Living with Coronary Heart Disease

A Johns Hopkins Press Health Book

Living with Coronary Heart Disease

A Guide for Patients and Families

Jerome E. Granato, M.D., F.A.C.C.

The Johns Hopkins University Press

Baltimore

Notes to the Reader
This book is not meant to substitute for medical care of people with heart disease, and treatment should not be based solely on its contents. Instead, treatment must be developed in a dialogue between the individual and his or her physician. This book has been written to help with that dialogue.

The author and publisher have made reasonable efforts to determine that the selection and dosage of drugs discussed in this text conform to the practices of the general medical community. The medications described do not necessarily have specific approval by the U.S. Food and Drug Administration for use in the diseases and dosages for which they are recommended. In view of ongoing research, changes in governmental regulations, and the constant flow of information relating to drug therapy and drug reactions, the reader is urged to check the package insert of each drug for any change in indications and dosage and for warnings and precautions. This is particularly important when the recommended agent is a new and/or infrequently used drug.

© 2008 The Johns Hopkins University Press
All rights reserved. Published 2008
Printed in the United States of America on acid-free paper
9 8 7 6 5 4 3 2 1

The Johns Hopkins University Press
2715 North Charles Street
Baltimore, Maryland 21218-4363
www.press.jhu.edu

Library of Congress Cataloging-in-Publication Data
Granato, Jerome E.
  Living with coronary heart disease : a guide for patients and families / Jerome E. Granato.
    p.   cm.
  ISBN-13: 978-0-8018-9024-6 (hardcover : alk. paper)
  ISBN-13: 978-0-8018-9025-3 (pbk. : alk. paper)
  ISBN-10: 0-8018-9024-1 (hardcover : alk. paper)
  ISBN-10: 0-8018-9025-X (pbk. : alk. paper)
  1. Coronary heart disease. 2. Coronary heart disease—Patients. I. Title.
  RC685.C6G72 2008
  616.1′23—dc22   2008006600

A catalog record for this book is available from the British Library.

Plates 1–9 are by Jacqueline Schaffer.

Special discounts are available for bulk purchases of this book. For more information, please contact Special Sales at 410-516-6936 or specialsales@press.jhu.edu.

The Johns Hopkins University Press uses environmentally friendly book materials, including recycled text paper that is composed of at least 30 percent post-consumer waste, whenever possible. All of our book papers are acid-free, and our jackets and covers are printed on paper with recycled content.

．．．

For

Dr. Joseph C. Alfenito, who inspired me to become a physician

Dr. Kenneth L. Baughman, who taught me to be both a student and a teacher

Dr. George A. Beller, who made me a cardiologist

And for my patients, who encouraged me to write this book

Contents

Color plates follow page 84.

Preface

....

In *Living with Coronary Heart Disease,* I accompany the reader on a journey where we encounter the symptoms, diagnostic process, and treatment options for this all-too-common condition. Along the way, my goal is to provide key insights that will enable you and your loved ones to make decisions based on knowledge and understanding. I hope that you will learn a lot. With the book now complete, I must admit that writing it was as much a journey for me as reading it will be for the reader. I learned a lot as well.

Writing this book was a labor of love that I thoroughly enjoyed and benefited from. Through this book I have become a better student, teacher, and physician. It forced me to think about what to say, how to say it, and why it should be said. Writing this book has not only taught me a lot about medicine, it has taught me much more. It reinforced my passion for the process of learning and teaching. It reminded me of how far scientific medicine has evolved, and how fortunate I am to be able to apply that knowledge in treating my patients. Our profession specializes in mothers and fathers, husbands and wives, brothers and sisters. It is a responsibility and a privilege that never grows old. This book was born of that belief.

In my journey in writing this book, I have had the opportunity to make many new friends and to reacquaint with many old ones. This too was an unanticipated joy of my journey. The list of those who have helped me along the way is long, and my thanks are heartfelt. While I have often thought of writing this book, I must thank one of my medical school classmates, Frank Mondimore, M.D., not only for convincing me to go ahead with my book project but also for introducing me to the wonderful people at the Johns Hopkins University Press.

I will never be able to find the right words to express the extent of my appreciation to Jacqueline Wehmueller, executive editor at the Johns Hopkins University Press. Throughout this journey, she has been both my compass and my captain, gently guiding me to this final destination. I, and the readers, have greatly benefited from her considerable talents. I am certain that this book could not have been completed without the efforts of Ashleigh McKown, assistant editor at the Johns Hopkins University Press. Ashleigh not only made sure that everything got done, she made sure that it got done correctly. Also at the Press, Kathy Alexander and the staff in marketing and publicity have done a wonderful job in making sure that this book gets in your hands. Many thanks to all of them.

While I take full responsibility for the content and style of the material presented in the book, my copyeditor, Melanie Mallon, has done a remarkable job of ensuring that my writing is lucid and grammatically correct. I still have much to learn, but with Melanie's oversight, I have become a better writer. *Living with Coronary Heart Disease* discusses complex medical topics in lay terms. These topics are often punctuated by beautiful illustrations. Throughout the book, you will see the medical art of Jacqueline Schaffer. Her extraordinary skill and keen insights help bring my words to life.

During my journey in writing this book, I discussed its concept and contents with many people. Special thanks go to Dr. Larry Gimple, Gerri Paulisick, and Tim Vismor for their many valuable comments and suggestions. This book could not have been written without my assistants, Judy Alabek and Annie Vamos. They have worked tirelessly to facilitate every aspect of my life, and in doing so, have allowed an author to emerge.

In writing this book, I am in debt to many but none more so than my wife, Judy, and my sons, Matthew and Timothy. They have been wildly enthusiastic about this book since its inception. I can never thank them enough, not only for their limitless affection and encouragement but also for their patience in enduring many hours of solitude while I embarked on my personal journey in writing *Living with Coronary Heart Disease*.

Introduction

....

If you are reading this book, chances are that either you or someone you know has coronary heart disease. This is a complicated disease, and understanding it can seem daunting, but nearly everyone
can become confident about and fully capable of living with coronary
heart disease. By talking with your doctors and reading this book
and other materials, you can become familiar with the causes and
symptoms of the disease, and with its treatments. You need to be an
active participant in making decisions about your treatment and your
health. *Living with Coronary Heart Disease: A Guide for Patients and
Families* will provide you with the information you need to become
an involved patient. It's a serious book for serious people who want
to thoroughly understand this complex medical condition.

In the pages of this book we will examine the spectrum of coronary heart disease, beginning with its chemical origins and ending
with how you can live a long and healthy life. We explore all the diagnostic tests, various medications, and therapeutic options. This book
takes you on a journey, as seen through the eyes of a typical patient,
addressing important questions as they might arise during the course
of an illness. We will build your knowledge base, layer upon layer,
until you truly understand what coronary heart disease is all about.

This book is not a substitute for your doctor's advice, care, or ex-
pertise. It is a book meant to help you work with your doctor. Actively
participating in your health care will be one of the most important
things you will ever do. Be prepared for it. Understand every aspect
of your condition and what will be required of you. Be comfortable
with the how and why of various treatment alternatives, and make
the choice that will be best for you. Take your time reading this book.
Discover how you can live fully with coronary heart disease.

ONE

What Is Coronary Heart Disease?

....

This book describes what coronary heart disease is and what causes it. It explains who is at risk for developing coronary heart disease and how the disease is recognized and diagnosed. And it describes in detail how coronary heart disease should be treated once it is diagnosed. With this information, you and your loved ones will be better prepared to actively participate with your health care providers in making some of the most important decisions you will ever face.

This chapter begins with the story of a middle-aged man named James. James's story illustrates several significant aspects of coronary heart disease. It also makes an important point: this disease affects many, many people, even men and women who try to do "all the right things" for their health. Unfortunately, this story could be your story or the story of someone you love.

James worked hard and had a good life, including a wife and three children—and a mortgage. He was thoughtful about his diet, and he exercised by doing chores around the house and yard. Like many people in his situation, he saw the doctor "when he was sick." To the best of his knowledge, he was a healthy man, enjoying his middle years. But James had indigestion that wouldn't go away. He took over-the-counter antacids, but he was still bothered by uncomfortable feelings in his chest. Finally, at the urging of his family, James went to see a doctor, who told him that he'd had a mild heart attack and that the indigestion was really something called angina pectoris. The symptoms he was experiencing were warning signs that another heart attack was possible. James was shocked to learn that he had coronary heart disease and that he needed urgent testing and treatment.

James couldn't believe this had happened to him. He had never been sick a day in his life and now, all of a sudden, he had heart disease.

After completing a stress test in which radioactive material was injected into his vein, James was scheduled to have a cardiac catheterization. James's doctor told him that he immediately needed to start taking several medications: platelet inhibitors, statin agents, beta-blocking drugs, and ACE inhibitors. His doctor also told him that he might need to have coronary angioplasty with stenting or, quite possibly, coronary bypass surgery. Understandably, James and his family were overwhelmed by this sudden diagnosis, all the medical tests, and the prospect of so many medications and procedures.

Many people find themselves in James's situation, not sure where to begin looking for answers to their questions. If you are reading this book, you may have many of the following concerns:

- How did this happen to me? My cholesterol level has always been good.
- What is a heart attack?
- Did I do something to cause this situation?
- How do I know that I really have coronary heart disease? How accurate are the medical tests?
- What are all these medications for? I hear they have side effects. Do I need to take them forever?
- Can't this condition be fixed with a balloon procedure?
- Do I have to have surgery? It sounds very dangerous.
- What is going to happen to me? How can I make sure that I don't have another heart attack?

All these questions are reasonable for someone who has been newly diagnosed with heart disease. In fact, men and women of all ages, races, and ethnic backgrounds who receive a diagnosis of heart disease ask these very same questions.

Who Gets Heart Disease?

In the United States, nearly one million people die from some form of *cardiovascular disease* (heart disease) every year. That's more than twenty-five hundred deaths per day, every day, day after day, month after month, and year after year. Cardiovascular disease is more lethal than any war or natural disaster. The economic, social and emotional burden of this disease on patients and their families is enormous. It influences every aspect of all of our lives. Not only scientists but also politicians, economists, and employers are concerned about the effect of this disease. Cardiovascular disease affects our grandparents and parents, our husbands and wives, our sisters and brothers, our relatives and our friends. We all know someone like James.

People tend to think of cardiovascular disease as something that elderly people get. Though it is most prevalent in people over the age of 65, cardiovascular disease affects many middle-age and even younger people. Many people also believe that heart disease affects mainly men. In fact, cardiovascular disease affects both men and women and all races (figure 1.1). It is a disease that knows no bounds.

One of the most important things to know about cardiovascular disease is that while the disease is not completely preventable, its course can be dramatically modified. Tremendous progress has been made in diagnosing and treating cardiovascular disease. Over the past thirty years, for example, the mortality rate from this disease has been cut in half. During this period, the average life expectancy in the United States has increased from 70.8 years to 77.9 years. This remarkable achievement is a result of the convergence of scientific discovery, technological development, and public education. As a society, we probably know more about cardiovascular disease than about any other condition.

The Cardiovascular Diseases

The term *cardiovascular disease*, which I have used until now, is too broad. Cardiovascular *diseases* actually comprise a host of disorders

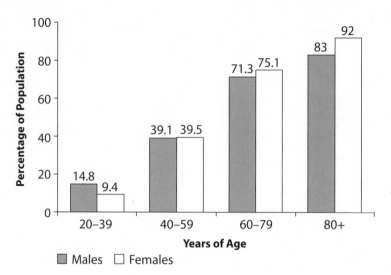

FIGURE 1.1. Prevalence of cardiovascular disease in Americans age 20 and older, by age and sex. Both men and women develop cardiovascular disease, and after age 60, a larger percentage of women than men have the disease. The disease is not limited to elderly people—adults of all ages develop cardiovascular disease. (*National Health and Nutrition Examination Study*, 1984–1994. Adapted and modified from American Heart Association, *Heart Disease and Stroke Statistics Update 2004.*)

that may involve numerous structures within the heart. The heart has structures similar to the pipes, valves, wires, and pistons in a car engine, all working together to pump blood through the body. Cardiovascular diseases can affect any or all of these parts and as a consequence impair the function of the heart. The cardiovascular diseases are divided into several different types based on the part of the heart affected. In 2004 there were 869,724 deaths attributed to cardiovascular disease in the United States. As you see in figure 1.2, coronary heart disease was by far the most prevalent cause, responsible for nearly half a million deaths.

Coronary heart disease is the process that damages the coronary arteries, which are among the most important structures in the heart (see plate 1). Continuing with the engine analogy, think of the coronary arteries as the pipes that bring the fuel supply to the engine. Coronary arteries bring blood to the heart muscle, supplying the heart

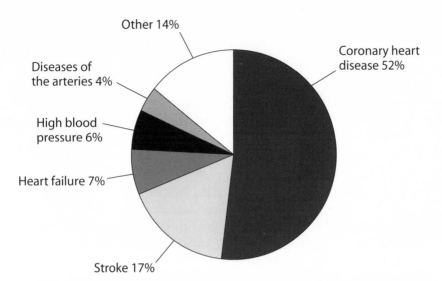

Other 14%

Coronary heart
disease 52%

Diseases of
the arteries 4%

High blood
pressure 6%

Heart failure 7%

Stroke 17%

FIGURE 1.2. Deaths from cardiovascular diseases in United States in 2004. There are many cardiovascular diseases. This figure illustrates the percentage of deaths from each kind of cardiovascular disease in the United States in 2004. Coronary heart disease is the most prevalent of the cardiovascular diseases. (Adapted and modified from American Heart Association, *Heart Disease and Stroke Statistics Update 2008*. Data from CDC/NCHS.)

with the oxygen and nutrients that enable it to function for many years. This book focuses on coronary heart disease, the disease that primarily affects these essential pipes—the coronary arteries—which extend from the aorta to and within the heart muscle.

As blood vessels go, the coronary arteries are rather small. At their origin at the aorta, these vessels measure only one to four millimeters in diameter. They then extend over the surface of the heart for another thirty to forty millimeters, branching into smaller and smaller vessels that extend deep into the heart muscle and deliver blood (and nutrients) to this vital organ. There are only three main coronary arteries supplying the entire heart. That's it. Just three pipes, barely a few millimeters in diameter, supplying the engine that keeps us alive. It is no wonder, then, that when these vessels become diseased, a portion of the heart becomes damaged.

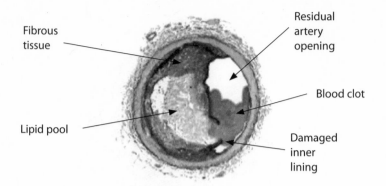

Fibrous tissue

Residual artery opening

Blood clot

Lipid pool

Damaged inner lining

FIGURE 1.3. Cross-sectional view of an atherosclerotic coronary artery. The figure demonstrates the complexity of an atherosclerotic plaque, inculding a large intravascular lipid pool, intravascular fibrous tissue, disruption of the endothelial lining, and an intravascular thrombus (or blood clot). (Still frame modified from an animation clip in the American College of Cardiology's *Self-Assessment Program V.*)

A Note on Terminology

Coronary heart disease is one of several cardiovascular diseases. Although I will primarily be using the term *coronary heart disease* in this book, coronary heart disease is known by several names. We have all heard "hardening of the arteries" used to describe the process that damages these important vessels. Sometimes it is referred to as "clogged arteries" or "plaque buildup."

The formal medical term for this process is *atherosclerosis* (ăth´-ə-rō-sklə-rō´-sĭs). Atherosclerosis comes from the Greek words for gruel, *athēra*, and hardening, *sklērōsis*. Atherosclerosis is a gruel-like hardening of the arteries. The hardening is the result of the arteries being "clogged" by the buildup of atherosclerotic "plaque." Thus:

atherosclerotic heart disease → coronary artery disease →
hardening of the arteries → plaque buildup

Moving from left to right in the sequence above, the general sentiment remains the same but the precision of the terms falls off. Coronary heart disease is a lay term used to describe the same process as the formal medical term atherosclerotic heart disease, or atherosclerosis. Figure 1.3 depicts a coronary artery that is partly obstructed by plaque. Coronary plaque is actually a complex structure comprising multiple components. *One key point to remember: what damages the coronary artery is a process that involves the inflammation, degeneration, and eventual thickening of the arterial wall.* It is not simply the buildup of sludge or debris inside the vessel. In fact, much of the coronary arterial damage occurs long before the artery is severely narrowed. This is why partly or minimally diseased blood vessels can suddenly become blocked by a clot.

Coronary heart disease is a *process* that involves the arteries throughout the body, damaging these vessels and thus limiting their ability to deliver blood to many organs, including the heart. It is a process that, to some degree, occurs in everyone. As a patient or a concerned loved one, you need to know as much about coronary heart disease as possible.

TWO

How Did This Happen?

Like James, many people respond to receiving a diagnosis of coronary heart disease by asking, "How did this happen to me?" Nearly everyone assumes that too much cholesterol is what causes coronary heart disease. Cholesterol has emerged as the villain, the entity identified as being responsible for the epidemic of coronary heart disease. In one sense, this is true. But while this reputation is well deserved, the fact is that cholesterol is not entirely bad. Cholesterol has many important functions in our body. Without cholesterol, we would not be able to live.

What's Cholesterol Got to Do with It?

Every cell in our body is encased in a protective covering, a cell membrane. This membrane is essential to cell life, acting as a protective barrier between the cell's inner machinery and the external world. Without cholesterol, these cell membranes would not have much structural integrity and would not hold together well. Without intact membranes, cells would break. Vital proteins would leak out of the cell, and the machinery that keeps us alive would fail. Our muscles would not contract, our nerves would not conduct electrical impulses, and our organs would not synthesize vital nutrients. Like the bricks and mortar of an industrial building, cholesterol helps protect our internal factories and power plants.

Cholesterol, however, is much more than a passive component of cellular makeup. It is an active ingredient in the synthesis of several important substances. Cholesterol is the precursor for all our sex hormones, for example. That's right. No cholesterol, no estrogen. No cholesterol, no testosterone. These and many other essential hormones begin as cholesterol, which is later modified at various sites within the body.

Cholesterol is also essential for the digestion of fats. It forms the basis of a series of compounds called *bile acids*. These important compounds are made in the liver and are secreted by the gallbladder after a meal. They allow us to absorb dietary fat from the digestive tract. Without bile acids, ingested fats would rapidly pass through our digestive tracts. We would have incessant diarrhea, develop vitamin deficiencies, and suffer from malnutrition. Simply put, we could not live without cholesterol. We need it to maintain our cellular structure, synthesize essential hormones, and absorb key nutrients from our diet.

Like everything in life, however, too much of a good thing can be a bad thing, and this is certainly the case with cholesterol. Learning to live with coronary heart disease means learning about cholesterol: what it is, where it comes from, and what it can do. This information helps you deal with cholesterol, as we all must do to be healthy, especially if we have coronary heart disease.

Many people think of cholesterol as a fat, but it isn't a fat at all. Cholesterol is actually a *sterol,* a compound with a chemical structure similar to alcohol. Cholesterol is composed of twenty-seven carbon atoms, forty-six hydrogen atoms, and one lonely oxygen atom. These atoms are linked together in an amazingly intricate pattern, giving rise to the compound we refer to as cholesterol. Cholesterol is made in the liver in a series of complex chemical reactions. One feature of cholesterol production that we need to understand is the concept of autoregulation.

Our bodies actually regulate how much cholesterol they make based on how much cholesterol they need and how much is available. Much as a thermostat regulates temperature, the liver monitors the body's cholesterol level and attempts to adjust it. If the cholesterol level is too low for your bodily needs, the liver senses the deficiency and begins to make more cholesterol. Once your cholesterol level rises to the appropriate level, the liver stops making cholesterol. The level to which our cholesterol is regulated varies from person to person and is determined by many factors, including bodily needs and genetic makeup. This system of autoregulation works quite well and is designed to ensure that our bodies never run out of this essential substance. Rest assured, you can never run out of cholesterol. Your liver has the capacity to make more than enough. This autoregulatory process would be nearly perfect if the liver were your only source of cholesterol. Unfortunately, it is not. Much of the cholesterol in your body is derived from cholesterol in your diet.

In Western societies, animal fat is a major source of energy, constituting 20 to 40 percent of caloric intake. Following a meal, dietary fat is broken into smaller molecules that coalesce to form large fat droplets. These fat droplets do not dissolve in water and thus cannot be absorbed by the cells lining our intestinal tract. For these fat droplets to be absorbed, they must first be broken down, or *emulsified,* in the intestine. This is done by combining the dietary fat droplets with a bile acid. As noted above, bile acids are produced by the liver and secreted by the gallbladder in response to a fatty meal. The emulsified (or dissolved) fats are then put into a "biological envelope" by the intestine in preparation for transport to the liver. The body makes many different types of biological envelopes to transport material to various locations. This particular biological envelope is called a *chylomicron.*

Chylomicrons are huge envelopes that contain the emulsified fats in the forms of triglycerides and cholesterol. They are the principle means of transporting dietary fat from the intestine to the liver. In the liver, chylomicrons are then disassembled, releasing their contents for reprocessing and repackaging in other envelopes for transport elsewhere in the body.

The biological envelopes that are made in the liver are different in that they are partly composed of proteins. They are often referred to as *lipoproteins.* Lipoproteins are the transport vehicles that carry cholesterol to numerous destinations throughout our body. Some lipoproteins are good for you, and some lipoproteins are bad. The chemical composition and the proportion of good and bad lipoproteins varies from person to person and are partly determined by genetic makeup. The nature of some lipoproteins can be modified through diet or medications, although this can be difficult (see chapters 4, 6, and 9).

After arriving at the liver, chylomicrons are degraded, and the cholesterol and triglycerides are reprocessed to form four broad categories of lipoproteins. They are *low density lipoproteins* (LDL), *high density lipoproteins* (HDL), *very light density lipoproteins* (VLDL), and *remnant lipoproteins*. Coronary heart disease is caused by an excess or deficiency of one or more of these lipoproteins. We will focus on LDL in this chapter.

Low density lipoproteins are often referred to as "bad cholesterol." They are the major means of cholesterol transport throughout the body. When an organ or tissue needs cholesterol for a specific purpose, it calls for LDL. The liver packages the cholesterol in an LDL envelope and sends it on its way via the bloodstream. Much of the LDL gets to its intended destination, but some LDL may get stuck along the way. As LDL particles travel through the bloodstream, some may adhere to the inner lining of blood vessel walls. The likelihood of an LDL particle sticking to a blood vessel wall depends on many factors, including the number of circulating LDL particles, their size, the nature of the protein forming the LDL envelope, and the condition of the blood vessel wall. Chapter 4 describes how common conditions like hypertension and diabetes, and lifestyle habits such as smoking, can affect each of these factors, thus increasing a person's risk of developing coronary heart disease.

Coronary Heart Disease Invades the Blood Vessel Wall

As noted in chapter 1, coronary heart disease is a process that affects the blood vessel wall. Contrary to popular belief, the formation of atherosclerotic plaque is not due to a buildup of cholesterol and debris inside the chamber of the blood vessel. Coronary heart disease is a degenerative and inflammatory process that begins *within the blood vessel wall*, causing it to weaken, enlarge, and eventually impair blood flow through the damaged artery.

The commonly used analogy that coronary heart disease is like leaves clogging a rain gutter is simply incorrect. Atherosclerotic plaque is more like a silently growing volcano than it is like debris in a rain gutter. This important distinction helps put treatment options in perspective. Recognizing that coronary heart disease is related to degeneration and inflammation of the blood vessel wall will help you understand how the successful treatment of coronary heart disease requires much more than simply lowering your cholesterol. The medical management of established coronary heart disease is discussed in chapters 6 and 7. For now, we need to examine in greater detail how the simple adhesion of an LDL molecule to the blood vessel wall ignites the atherosclerotic process.

Coronary arteries are pretty amazing structures. They supply large volumes of blood to your heart in an uninterrupted manner for years on end. The blood vessels are under high pressure, yet they flex and expand with each heartbeat. They are incredibly dynamic, efficiently responding to your heart's needs on a moment's notice. For example, if your heart requires more blood during exercise, the coronary arteries automatically enlarge to increase the blood supply to this vigorously beating muscle. When the situation changes, these vessels instantly change size again, facilitating efficient use of the energy they supply.

Normal coronary arteries are able to react to a large variety of stimuli to ensure that your heart continues to receive all the blood it needs. They are far more than just passive pipes that carry blood to the heart. They are complex, living structures that react and accommodate to the ever-changing demands of your internal engine. It is important to remember that this is how normal coronary arteries work. When the atherosclerotic process invades the blood vessel, the artery's ability to react and fulfill these important functions becomes impaired. Unfortunately, this arterial invasion can begin long before you have any symptoms of heart disease. How can someone whose cholesterol has "always been good" get coronary heart disease? The answer lies in understanding the nature of the blood vessel wall.

A Hose and Much More

In some ways, a coronary artery is like a garden hose, a flexible, multilayered pipe transporting a liquid at high pressure. The healthy coronary artery can be divided into three key layers. These are depicted in part A of plate 2.

The outmost layer of an artery is called the *adventitia*. Made of fibrous tissue, this outer layer gives the artery the strength to withstand high pressure. Picture it as steel reinforcement for the hose. The middle layer of the artery is called the *media*. This layer is rich with smooth muscle cells that are arranged in an orderly and circumferential manner. These smooth muscles cells are very much alive and working. When our blood vessels need to enlarge to accommodate more blood flow, the muscle cells in the media relax and allow the vessel to dilate. If the blood pressure should fall too low, the muscle cells in the media contract, causing the vessel to constrict, narrowing the artery to ensure an adequate blood pressure and blood flow. The muscle cells in the media are so important in regulating blood flow that they are able to replicate and grow should they become damaged. This protective mechanism can go awry in someone with coronary heart disease, fueling the formation of atherosclerotic plaque.

The innermost layer of the coronary artery is called the *intima*. This intimal layer is actually a lining of specialized cells called *endothelium*. This endothelial lining may be only one or two cells thick, but it is unquestionably the most important part of the blood vessel. The endothelium lines every inch of the inside of our blood vessels. It forms a protective coating that shields the media from the many toxins that may circulate in the blood. The intima, however, is far more than a passive protective lining. Like the media, it is very much alive and actively participates in maintaining the health of the blood vessel.

The Importance of the Endothelial Lining

The endothelial cells, forming the intimal layer, produce several important substances that ensure our blood cells won't stick to the inside of the blood vessel. Analogous to a Teflon lining, endothelial cells also produce other substances that assist in the control of vascular tone, helping the media to dilate or constrict as needed. When the endothelial lining is damaged, these functions become impaired. A damaged endothelial lining can become "sticky," allowing unwanted toxins to adhere to its surface. With a damaged endothelium, the coronary artery's protective barrier has been breached. This allows toxins that circulate in our blood to infiltrate the blood vessel wall and take up residence in what was a pristine media. LDL is one of those toxins that can adhere to and eventually penetrate the endothelial layer.

The atherosclerotic process begins when LDL penetrates the endothelium, enters the blood vessel wall, and wreaks havoc with the all-important muscle cells residing in the media. With damaged endothelial and media layers, the artery's ability to regulate blood pressure and blood flow also becomes impaired. What was once a living and dynamic conduit starts to become a rigid pipe. Let's look at this sequence of events in greater detail.

What's So Bad about LDL Cholesterol?

Recall that LDL is the body's transport envelope for cholesterol. LDL particles circulate through the bloodstream to deliver cholesterol to sites that require the many essential functions described earlier. Some of these LDL particles, however, can stick to the endothelium that lines the blood vessels. When there are many LDL particles circulating in our bloodstream, they tend to clump together, covering the endothelium like condensation on a shower door. Unfortunately, the endothelium can leak, and some of the LDL particles may seep through this protective lining and penetrate the blood vessel wall. This is depicted in plate 2B. How and why this occurs is the subject of intense investigation. One thing is clear. The more circulating LDL particles there are in your blood (i.e., the higher your measured LDL level), the more likely it is that an LDL particle will penetrate the endothelial lining and initiate the atherosclerotic process.

LDL particles are composed differently in different people. In some people, the proteins forming the LDL envelope may make it easier for LDL to penetrate the intima. In others, proteins that form the LDL envelope may hinder the process of LDL penetration. The protein composition of the LDL envelope is partly determined by genetics. Not all LDL is alike. This may explain why some people have rather high LDL levels and do not have coronary heart disease, while others have only mild elevations of LDL but have advanced atherosclerotic disease. Some conditions (such as diabetes) may make a person more susceptible to developing coronary heart disease by altering the composition of LDL so that it is more likely to penetrate the endothelium. Other behaviors and conditions (like tobacco use and hypertension) may damage the endothelial surface, enhancing the ability of LDL to penetrate this protective barrier. The migration of LDL into the arterial wall is only the beginning of the destructive process we call coronary heart disease. Subintimal LDL (LDL that has penetrated the intimal layer) is the biological equivalent of a Trojan horse. Once LDL has penetrated the arterial wall, the villains hastily shed their disguise and call for more destructive reinforcements.

The Arrival of Vascular Inflammation

Once inside the blood vessel wall, the LDL envelope is quickly opened; the LDL is then transformed to a more active state. This active state is referred to as *modified LDL*. Modified LDL acts like a beacon, sending out a series of chemical signals that call for another essential contributor to coronary heart disease—inflammation. Modified LDL stimulates the endothelium lining of the blood vessel, causing it to release a number of proteins that attract white blood cells to the region. The newly stimulated endothelial lining then grows adhesion molecules on its surface. These molecules essentially act like Velcro strips in the blood vessel channel by latching on to circulating white blood cells and pulling them into the blood vessel wall. The addition of white blood cells to the composition of the blood vessel wall is an essential step in the atherosclerotic process. These cells transform a process that began as an accumulation of cholesterol into a process of inflammation. Inflammation causes swelling, irritation, and injury. The atherosclerotic process involves all of this and more.

Vascular adhesion molecules (the Velcro) on the endothelial cells latch on to a specific type of white blood cell called a *monocyte*. Like fish on a hook, monocytes are gradually pulled into the blood vessel wall. Once inside the blood vessel wall, the monocyte transforms into a *macrophage*. Macrophages eat things; these specific macrophages soon feast on all the readily available modified LDL in the blood vessel wall. The macrophages become "lipid laden," gorging themselves on the now abundant intra-arterial LDL. This lipid-laden feast is depicted in plate 2B.

Lipid-laden macrophages can become quite large and are often called *foam cells*. They constitute the bulk of the intra-arterial gruel that forms the atherosclerotic plaque. The atherosclerotic plaque, however, contains more than foam cells. We have all heard the expression misery loves company. Such is the case with foam cells. These intra-arterial cesspools also signal and stimulate smooth muscle cells to migrate from the adjacent media layer. The smooth muscle cells begin to replicate and congregate just below the endothelial surface. An intra-arterial "pimple," called a *fibrous cap*, forms, containing a collection of lipid-laden macrophages and debris that now constitute an atherosclerotic plaque, as shown in plate 2B.

Cholesterol (in the form of LDL particles) plays a major role in initiating the atherosclerotic process. The atherosclerotic plaque itself, however, is composed of lipid-laden macrophages, smooth muscle cells, and other debris that now reside *inside the wall* of the coronary artery, as illustrated in plate 2B. Note that a rather large atherosclerotic plaque has formed a very thick blood vessel wall, but despite these dramatic changes in the blood vessel wall, there has been relatively little narrowing of the actual blood vessel channel. The atherosclerotic process has actually *remodeled* the coronary artery, causing it to expand so that most of the plaque bulges outward and away from the blood vessel channel, thickening the wall but actually compromising the blood vessel channel to a lesser degree.

Plate 2B helps illustrate that the atherosclerotic plaque obstructing the blood vessel chamber is only the tip of the iceberg. A slowly expanding atherosclerotic plaque can remodel the coronary artery without any disruption in blood flow. It can grow and grow for many years, gradually infiltrating the blood vessel without causing any symptoms. Coronary artery remodeling is the camouflage that masks growth of atherosclerotic plaque.

You now know how James developed coronary heart disease. His current health problems reflect an atherosclerotic process that has been silently present for quite some time. This process affects millions of people worldwide. Coronary heart disease, or atherosclerosis, is a complex series of events that, while initiated by cholesterol products, actually involves much more. Coronary heart disease involves vascular adhesion molecules, white blood cells, lipid-laden macrophages, smooth muscle proliferation, and vascular remodeling. Coronary heart disease isn't as much about the buildup of debris as it is about damage to the coronary artery's endothelial lining, the inflammatory response, and the subsequent destruction of the blood vessel wall. This is a very important concept that will reappear throughout this book in discussions about how to direct therapies against atherosclerosis.

The story of the atherosclerotic process to be told here is not yet complete, however. We need to ask another question: How does the quiescent atherosclerotic plaque eventually make its presence known? It can occur with great fanfare, or it can be ignored. It is time to find out what a heart attack is.

THREE

What Is a Heart Attack?

....

James could not believe the news. How could he have had a heart attack? He had never been taken by ambulance to an emergency room because of a heart attack. Isn't that how you knew that you'd had one? James could not remember even having chest pain. Aside from some occasional indigestion, he felt well. Like many people, he thought a heart attack was a dramatic event. The reality, however, is that not all heart attacks "hurt." Like James, many people are told they have had a mild heart attack, and they may take comfort in the word "mild." Unfortunately, it is false comfort. This chapter describes exactly what a heart attack is and explains how untamed coronary heart disease may cause someone to have a heart attack.

Heart attack is the lay term often used to describe a *myocardial infarction,* which is the medical term that describes the irreversible loss of cardiac muscle. Myocardial (mī´-ō-kär´-dē-al) is another word for heart tissue. Infarction (ĭn-färk´-shən) means tissue death or destruction. A myocardial infarction can be small or large. It can arrive with unmistakable symptoms or it can masquerade as a common malady, largely ignored by the person experiencing it. A myocardial infarction can involve a critical part of the heart, causing great disability, or it can be localized to an area of lesser importance, arriving with barely a whimper. In any case, a myocardial infarction represents the loss of a precious personal asset—cardiac muscle. It can never be taken lightly. Learning to live with coronary heart disease means understanding how the atherosclerotic process can lead to a myocardial infarction.

A myocardial infarction is a sentinel event. It demands your attention. If it happened once, it can surely happen again, with a decidedly different outcome. Consider these statistics from the American Heart Association:

- Within six years after a first heart attack, 18 percent of men and 35 percent of women will have a *second* heart attack.
- Nearly 7 percent of people who have a heart attack will die suddenly, before they can reach a hospital.
- Of the people who survive their first heart attack, 22 percent of men and 46 percent of women will develop disabling congestive heart failure. Almost 10 percent of people who survive their first heart attack will eventually have a stroke.

As these statistics indicate, a heart attack, big or small, identifies you as being at risk for several adverse events. Happily, the number of heart attacks and deaths from heart attacks is declining each year because of specific therapies aimed at treating the cause of these life-threatening events. All these therapies work by balancing a mismatch between the coronary artery blood supply and the heart's demand for oxygen.

Cardiovascular Accounting: Balancing Oxygen Supply and Demand

Like any muscle in the body, the heart requires a reliable and plentiful blood supply, bringing with it a continuous stream of oxygen and other nutrients. With exercise, the heart's demand for these nutrients increases. The coronary arteries supplying the heart respond to this demand by increasing the flow of blood. Normal coronary arteries respond to the heart's demand for more blood by dilating to the point where the blood flow can increase as much as fivefold. This ability to augment coronary blood flow is referred to as the *vasodilator response*. In coronary arteries that have been affected by the atherosclerotic process, this vasodilator response is impaired or absent.

To understand how this restricted blood flow impairs the heart's functioning, think about how your car would perform if it could not increase its fuel supply when you stepped on the accelerator. In atherosclerotic coronary arteries, this defect in vascular control sets the stage for an imbalance to occur between the oxygen demanded by the heart and the oxygen that is supplied. In the heart, if the oxygen demand exceeds the oxygen supply (for example, during exercise), the heart muscle effectively suffocates and begins to malfunction. This condition of myocardial suffocation and malfunction is referred to as *myocardial ischemia* (ĭ-skē´-mē-ə).

The symptoms of myocardial ischemia vary. The most common symptom is discomfort. If you have narrowed coronary arteries and overexert yourself (oxygen demand exceeds oxygen supply), you may experience discomfort. "Discomfort" is a much better term than "pain" when describing the symptoms of ischemia. Patients describe this discomfort as being more like heaviness, a squeezing or a dull ache, rather than true pain. This chest discomfort is frequently brought on by physical exertion. Effort-induced discomfort is called *angina pectoris* (ăn-jī´-nə pek´-tər-ĭs). Angina pectoris may be the early warning sign of an impending heart attack and *must not be ignored.*

The discomfort of angina pectoris is not necessarily located in the chest. This sensation can occur in the arms, shoulders, back, or jaw. It isn't necessarily dramatic, either, and can easily be misinterpreted or attributed to some other process. James thought he had indigestion. Other people may conclude that they pulled a muscle. Myocardial ischemia usually produces some form of discomfort. It is important to pay attention to this feeling. Prolonged discomfort of any type, or any repeated symptom of discomfort, requires medical attention.

A pump without a sufficient fuel supply can't work very well. Another way myocardial ischemia may make itself known is by impairing the contraction of the cardiac muscle itself. Inefficient cardiac contraction leads to shortness of breath, and shortness of breath is frequently, but not always, accompanied by chest discomfort. It is sometimes easy to mistakenly blame effort-related shortness of breath on being out of shape, on tackling too steep a hill, or on cold weather. In many ways, effort-related shortness of breath is more worrisome than angina pectoris, for it implies that there is a significant alteration of cardiac pumping with exercise. *Pay attention to the symptom of effort-related shortness of breath.* Take it seriously. Learning to live with coronary heart disease requires recognizing the various ways in which myocardial ischemia makes itself known, and promptly seeing a doctor.

Not only may an ischemic heart muscle contract poorly, it may also conduct electrical impulses abnormally. Clinical *signs* (what the doctor finds on examination) of impaired electrical activity in the heart include an irregular heartbeat and specific changes in the electrocardiogram (EKG, or ECG) pattern. Patients may experience *symptoms* such as an irregular heartbeat as palpitations, commonly described as a thumping sensation in the chest. (Symptoms are what the patient experiences, and *presenting symptoms* is doctor-speak for what brings a person to visit a doctor in the first place.) With palpitations, the extra heartbeats pound more vigorously and become noticeable (palpable) to the patient. They can be frightening. An EKG measures the electrical activity of the heart with each beat. It is an important test for people with coronary heart disease. When the heart muscle is ischemic or permanently damaged, its pattern of electrical activity may be altered. This change may be reflected in a new and abnormal pattern in the EKG. Even though James was not aware of having had a heart attack, his EKG was abnormal. Because James's heart was now conducting electrical impulses differently from the way it had in the past, his doctor was able to surmise that his heart had been injured and to decide that further testing was needed.

Taken alone or in combination, symptoms of chest discomfort, shortness of breath, or palpitations may indicate a critical imbalance between the heart's oxygen supply and its demand. Myocardial ischemia showing up as any of these symptoms strongly suggests that coronary blood flow has been limited by the atherosclerotic process. The good news about myocardial ischemia is that it goes away. Stop exercising and the symptoms subside. Take some nitroglycerin under your tongue (medically balancing the supply-demand mismatch) and the symptoms go away. Don't be fooled by the temporary nature of these symptoms or how easily you can make them go away. They are indicative of a real and potentially dangerous underlying disorder. They suggest that your coronary arteries are critically narrowed and are limiting the blood flow that is vital to your heart's function. Experiencing recurring symptoms of myocardial ischemia and not getting medical advice and treatment is like wiping up a puddle on the floor and not investigating its source on the roof. Left untreated, myocardial ischemia will keep coming back and ultimately may represent a more dangerous situation—a myocardial infarction.

Myocardial ischemia goes hand in hand with coronary arteries that have been significantly narrowed by the atherosclerotic process described in chapter 2. A myocardial infarction occurs when one of these arteries is suddenly and completely blocked, depriving the heart of oxygen. Atherosclerotic plaque is the basis of the coronary occlusion. The transition between a stable, nonocclusive plaque and an unstable one signals the completion of the atherosclerotic process.

Developing an Unstable Atherosclerotic Plaque

As discussed in chapter 1, coronary heart disease is much more than simple "hardening" of the arteries. It is a process characterized by degeneration and inflammation of the arterial wall. As the lipid-laden macrophages and smooth muscle cells accumulate beneath the endothelial lining, they produce various toxic substances that contribute to the death of the cells. The atherosclerotic plaque that results is a collection of foam cells and cellular debris that tend to coalesce and form a soft lipid pool just below the endothelial lining. The stimulated smooth muscle cells tend to migrate toward the endothelial surface of the plaque, forming a dome, the fibrous cap, that surrounds the lipid-laden foam cells (plate 3).

The fibrous cap is a protective barrier between the enlarging lipid pool and the blood channel. As the atherosclerotic process continues, white blood cells and toxic substances continue to accumulate within the plaque, inflaming the surrounding tissue and accelerating the destructive process beneath the fibrous cap. Eventually the toxins produced by the ongoing inflammatory process may cause the plaque's fibrous cap to rupture, exposing the accumulated atherosclerotic debris to the blood. In many ways, the atherosclerotic plaque has grown like a volcano and has suddenly erupted. The blood vessel that once had a smooth endothelial surface now has a large ulcerated crater.

After the rupture, the exposed atherosclerotic debris contains a substance known as *tissue factor*. Tissue factor acts like glue for *fibrin* and platelets circulating in the blood. Fibrin consists of thin strands of protein that accumulate at the site of injury. These fibrin strands cling together, much like a net, trapping platelets and other materials on the rapidly growing *thrombus*, or blood clot. The interaction between tissue factor, fibrin, and platelets causes a thrombus to quickly form over the ruptured fibrous cap (plate 3), much like a scab over an open wound. If the thrombus is large enough, the coronary artery becomes completely obstructed and a myocardial infarction begins to evolve. If the fibrous cap rupture is small, a partially obstructive thrombus may form, causing intermittent coronary obstruction and *unstable* angina symptoms. The situation is unstable because the partially occlusive clot, producing intermittent symptoms, can easily and swiftly progress to a full myocardial infarction.

There's No Such Thing as a Mild Heart Attack

You may have known someone who had a "mild" heart attack. Chances are they were describing a myocardial infarction produced by a partially occlusive thrombus. As noted above, myocardial ischemia will disrupt the heart's electrical activity, and this disruption may be observed on the EKG. James's doctor observed this change in James's EKG and concluded that James had had a heart attack. The magnitude of the electrical disruption is used to hypothesize whether a person has a complete coronary artery occlusion or a partial coronary artery occlusion. The electrical disruption involves a portion of the EKG known as the *ST segment*. A myocardial infarction produced by a fully occlusive thrombus is referred to as *ST-elevation myocardial infarction* (STEMI), and one produced by a partially occlusive thrombus is referred to as *non-ST-elevation myocardial infarction* (NSTEMI).

It is common to refer to a STEMI as a major heart attack and an NSTEMI as a mild one, but there is nothing mild about any type of myocardial infarction. Consider that

- both types of myocardial infarction are caused by the same atherosclerotic process;
- both types involve plaque rupture and coronary thrombosis;
- both types irreversibly damage heart muscle;
- both types can cause death; and
- both types require aggressive early management.

The only difference between these two significant events is the initial therapeutic approach.

It would be natural to assume that a myocardial infarction caused by an incomplete coronary thrombus (an NSTEMI) is preferable to a myocardial infarction caused by a larger and more permanent blood clot (a STEMI). This assumption, however, is completely wrong. Over time, an NSTEMI left untreated carries a risk of mortality that is actually higher than that of a STEMI. How can this be? Thinking about the origins of a myocardial infarction, we can see that an NSTEMI is actually an "incomplete heart attack." While the partially and intermittently occlusive blood clot has initially caused only a mild amount of cardiac damage, the situation is unstable. The ruptured fibrous cap persists. The intracoronary blood clot remains adherent to the blood vessel wall, slowly growing. This intermittent and partial occlusion may continue until the vessel completely reoccludes later with much more damaging results. Left unchecked, NSTEMIs frequently progress to STEMIs over time.

Mild heart attacks, or NSTEMIs, must be taken seriously. Over the past twenty years, the National Institutes of Health has sponsored a series of clinical studies referred to as the Thrombolysis in Myocardial Infarction (TIMI) trials. These clinical trials have been enormously helpful in understanding how to treat patients with myocardial infarctions. One of the most valuable insights from the TIMI trials has been the emergence of the TIMI risk score. Using the TIMI risk score, a doctor can accurately estimate the risk of a second serious cardiac event following the initial NSTEMI. Figure 3.1 depicts the risk for death, repeat myocardial infarction, or symptoms worsening to the point where an emergency procedure is required in patients with a recent NSTEMI.

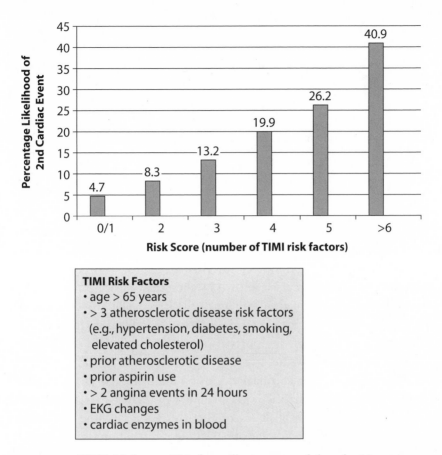

FIGURE 3.1. TIMI risk factors. This figure illustrates a tool that physicians use to calculate a patient's risk of having an adverse event, considering the patient's specific risk factors and clinical situation. (Adapted from Elliott M. Antman et al., "The TIMI Risk Score for Unstable Angina/Non-ST-Elevation MI: A Method for Prognostication and Therapeutic Decision Making," *Journal of the American Medical Association* 284 (2000): 835–42.)

Let's try to put into perspective what the TIMI risk score tells us. Assume that you have just had a mild heart attack (NSTEMI). Further, you are a 66-year-old smoker with hypertension, high cholesterol, and diabetes who had this attack while taking aspirin. You have had two episodes of angina pectoris in the past day. In this setting, the risk of a second cardiac event (including death) during the next two weeks is over 25 percent. One in four patients with a similar risk factor profile and a mild heart attack will die, have a second heart attack, or require an emergency intervention within two weeks of their initial presentation. This is one reason why there can be little comfort in having "only" a mild heart attack. Having a mild heart attack, or NSTEMI, identifies you as someone with active and unstable atherosclerotic plaque. You have a problem that needs to be dealt with. The good news is that many forms of treatment will significantly reduce the risk of repeat myocardial infarction (see chapters 6, 7, and 8). With proper treatment, potentially everyone with an NSTEMI can be heart healthy.

While an untreated NSTEMI may be followed by worsening angina symptoms or a repeat myocardial infarction, a STEMI has an entirely different course. Here, the coronary artery has been completely obstructed by a blood clot. As discussed previously, this blockage may initially make itself known by chest discomfort, poor cardiac contraction, or electrical instability of the heart. The heart muscle is completely deprived of its essential nutrients, and it is suffocating. If this process continues, the portion of the heart supplied by the occluded vessel begins to die. Irreversible muscle damage begins as early as forty minutes after coronary occlusion and is largely complete six hours later. Thus, there is a very small window of opportunity to disrupt the clot, reestablish essential coronary blood flow, and save cardiac muscle. There are various possible interventions, each bringing a significant improvement in patient survival (see chapters 6 and 7). *The damage of a myocardial infarction can be minimized if treated early.* If you think you are having a myocardial infarction, you must seek emergency medical attention.

The Consequences of a Heart Attack

When cardiac muscle has been damaged, the damage is irreversible. Cardiac tissue, unlike skin, bone, or other tissue, does not regenerate. The damaged cardiac tissue goes on to form scar tissue, and the formation of cardiac scar tissue has several consequences. Cardiac scars do not contract, so the development of cardiac scar tissue permanently reduces the contracting ability of the heart. If you have had an ST-elevation myocardial infarction, you have lost some cardiac horsepower. Depending on the size of the scar and its location in the heart, this loss of power can be significant.

Initially, when a portion of the heart becomes damaged, the other previously unaffected portions of the heart begin to work harder. Picture a racing scull. If one of the rowers drops out, those remaining need to row harder. The same is true with your heart. A compensatory increase in the vigor of muscle contraction ensures that your heart pumps enough blood to continue to meet the demands of the body. Like any muscle that is exercised, this now overworked heart muscle undergoes some alteration. It begins to thicken, or *hypertrophy*. Initially this hypertrophy is good, because it enables the heart to continue pumping blood throughout the body. Over time, however, this abnormal thickening of the heart is bad. The thickened muscle becomes stiff, causing the pressure within the heart to rise.

Pause and think about what is happening here. If you have a heart attack damaging one portion of your heart, a previously normal and totally separate portion of your heart will, after time, start to change and eventually malfunction as well. While the previously normal portion of the heart thickens, the damaged portion of the heart also changes. The damaged tissue is replaced by scar tissue, and this newly formed scar tissue may also cause problems. The scarred portion of your heart is a weakness in the heart's wall and acts like a bubble on an automobile tire. In response to higher pressure within your heart, the scar tissue begins to expand. This *infarct expansion* causes your heart to enlarge. Following a STEMI, the heart not only contracts poorly, it becomes stiffer (due to hypertrophy of the normal area) and enlarged (due to expansion of the infarcted area). This process of infarct expansion and compensatory cardiac thickening is referred to as *cardiac remodeling* (see plate 4).

Cardiac remodeling has adverse clinical consequences for the patient and is responsible for many of the frightening statistics referred to in the beginning of this chapter. Cardiac remodeling explains why patients who have survived a STEMI develop an enlarged heart and a tendency to accumulate fluid in their lungs. This condition is called *congestive heart failure*. Cardiac remodeling also allows blood to pool within the heart, which facilitates the formation of blood clots within the main pumping chamber. These clots may break, resulting in a stroke. Further, cardiac remodeling alters the electrical pathways inside the heart, which sets the stage for the heart to become irritable, quite possibly culminating in a *fatal arrhythmia*. An arrhythmia is any alteration in the transmission of electrical signals through the heart. The presence of scar tissue can disrupt this transmission to the point that the heart beats far too fast or beats chaotically (fibrillation). When this occurs, the heart muscle can no longer contract, resulting in death. Death from heart attack is almost always the result of arrhythmia.

Cardiac remodeling represents the aftershocks of the original earthquake that was your myocardial infarction. Cardiac remodeling is a predictable consequence of STEMI. Surviving the initial damage of a myocardial infarction is not enough. Long-term survival is dependent on aggressive treatment of the adverse consequences of cardiac remodeling. In particular, reducing the extent of remodeling reduces your future risk for congestive heart failure, stroke, and death. This treatment is discussed in chapter 6. Before turning to treatment, however, we'll take a closer look at what causes coronary heart disease and how it is diagnosed.

Coronary heart disease is a process that involves much more than having an excess of cholesterol in the blood. The interaction between blood vessel inflammation, proliferation of smooth muscle cells, and blood clot formation is equally important in the atherosclerotic process. If you already have coronary heart disease, you need to tame it—before you develop symptoms. We now turn to ways in which you can take charge of the atherosclerotic process.

FOUR

Did I Do Something to Cause This?

Understandably, people who are diagnosed with coronary heart disease wonder whether they did something to cause their disease. There is no simple answer to this question. Many risk factors make a person more likely to develop coronary heart disease. Some of these risk factors can be modified, while others cannot. Some people have done things that contributed to their heart problem, and other people have not. Learning to live with coronary heart disease means learning to identify and modify these risk factors.

Many of the risk factors for coronary heart disease are well known to most Americans because our doctors and the American Heart Association have done a remarkable job of educating us about these risks (see table 4.1). In this chapter, we will review how much each of these risk factors contributes to coronary heart disease.

Understanding Risk Factors for Coronary Heart Disease

Don't we all wish we could avoid getting old? Advanced age is a major risk factor for developing coronary heart disease. Much like gray hair and wrinkles, all of us will eventually develop some degree of athero- sclerotic, or coronary heart, disease. It is the manifestation of wear and tear on the blood vessels that normally comes with aging. Because the incidence of coronary heart disease increases with advancing age, advanced age is an important risk factor for the development of this disease. Unfortunately, we can't do much about aging. While nearly

TABLE 4.1 *Risk Factors for Coronary Heart Disease*

---

advanced age
elevated LDL cholesterol level (>130)
reduced HDL cholesterol level (<40)
family history of premature coronary heart disease
male gender
diabetes
hypertension
tobacco use
obesity

Source: Adapted from the American Heart Association's *Heart Disease and Stroke Statistics Update 2008.*

everyone develops some degree of coronary heart disease, people can control the extent to which this disease becomes a problem for them.

Chapter 2 described the role of cholesterol in the formation of atherosclerotic plaque. Cholesterol is an essential ingredient of coronary heart disease. While there may be some variation in the relationship between cholesterol and this disease among individuals, there is little question that in general, higher levels of LDL cholesterol are associated with a higher incidence of coronary heart disease. The more atherosclerosis you have, the more likely you are to suffer from its consequences in the form of a heart attack, stroke, and ultimately death. Researchers have looked at the relationship between cholesterol levels and cardiac-related mortality in Asia, Europe, and North America. They found that while countries vary in the amount of cholesterol in their diets, the relationship between cholesterol and cardiac-related mortality is clear. The higher the serum cholesterol level, the greater the risk of death from complications of coronary heart disease. The relationship between death from cardiovascular disease and elevated cholesterol levels is so strong that the treatment of elevated cholesterol levels is one of the major public health thrusts of modern medicine.

Many factors help determine an individual's cholesterol level. There is little question that a healthy diet has a favorable effect on body weight, cholesterol levels, and, ultimately, cardiovascular risk. Much of the variation in cholesterol levels between countries can be attributed to dietary variations in the consumption of saturated fats and cholesterol. Not surprisingly, the United States and Northern European populations, which have diets that are rich in saturated fats, have a much higher average cholesterol level and a much higher cardiovascular mortality than Asian populations. Saturated fats are among the most unhealthy of foods. Derived principally from animal fats, saturated fats are the primary dietary source of LDL cholesterol.

There are many excellent ways for you to eat better for your heart's health. The basic principle is to minimize the proportion of daily calories you obtain from fat, especially saturated fat. The National Cholesterol Education Program (NCEP) is an excellent resource for information about heart healthy diets. The current NCEP recommendations suggest a diet in which 25 to 35 percent of calories are obtained from fat, and only 7 percent (or less) of these calories are derived from saturated fat. This is no easy feat. For example, many fast foods provide 30 to 50 percent of the daily caloric requirements from fat, and 15 to 30 percent of these calories come from saturated fats.

Diets rich in fish, fruits, complex carbohydrates (bran, oatmeal, brown rice), and vegetables have been shown to reduce the risk of coronary heart disease. This is why there is a low risk of cardiovascular death in Mediterranean and Asian countries relative to Western countries. Recent studies indicate that adhering to the NCEP Step II diet will result in a decline of approximately 20 percent in both total and LDL cholesterol. This reduction in cholesterol certainly reduces the risk of coronary heart disease, but is it enough of a reduction for someone who may be genetically prone to develop heart disease? Answering this question involves reviewing some of the large clinical research trials testing the effects of various cholesterol-lowering agents. Before doing that, let me describe how clinical research trials are conducted.

The Importance of Clinical Research Trials

Good science is based on facts. This concept, in the context of medicine, is sometimes referred to as evidence-based medicine, in which the evidence is usually the summation of scientific data accumulated via the *prospective, randomized, placebo-controlled, double-blind* trial. Let's take a look at each of these terms.

For a clinical research trial to have maximum validity, it must be *prospective,* meaning "looking forward." In planning a clinical research trial, the investigators must formulate an educated guess (called a *hypothesis*) about what they expect the study to show. A clinical research trial, then, is a test designed to prove or disprove the hypothesis. By being *prospective,* the study's relevant clinical information (age, for example) is identified at the beginning of the trial. This information is then collected on all subjects, moving forward, on an ongoing basis. This type of trial usually avoids the bias of looking at a preexisting pool of data (called a *retrospective* analysis) and allowing the investigator to pick and choose data or possibly view the information in light of some preconceived outcome.

When comparing two types of treatments, prospective patients must receive the treatment in a completely *randomly assigned* manner. The investigators should not be able to choose who does and who does not get a specific therapy. Each therapeutic option must be equally likely to be given to all patients. This avoids the possibility of bias being introduced by, for example, the very ill patients getting one form of treatment and healthier patients getting another.

In evaluating a specific treatment, it is important to be able to compare the clinical *course* (outcome) of patients receiving treatment to the clinical course of patients in the trial who were not receiving treatment. The use of a *placebo control* gives the investigators a fair standard of comparison for the new treatment. Some participants in the trial receive treatment, and some participants receive a placebo (either a nontherapeutic treatment or the standard treatment). Last, if at all possible, the study should be *double-blind,* meaning that neither the investigators nor the patients know whether they are receiving a placebo or the treatment under investigation. This type of blinding is essential in eliminating bias brought about by knowing which patients received a specific therapy. Prospective, randomized, double-blind, placebo-controlled clinical research trials are difficult to design and execute. Nonetheless, they can provide convincing answers to important clinical questions. This type of clinical research forms the basis for some of our most important therapeutic decisions.

All patients participating in this type of clinical research must be fully informed of the randomized, double-blinded, and placebo-controlled nature of the study as well as the potential risks and benefits of their participation. Their *informed consent* is required before they enroll. (Informed consent involves obtaining the participants' signature on a form stating that the trial has been thoroughly explained to them.) All prospective, randomized, double-blind, placebo-controlled clinical research trials are closely monitored by two entities designed to protect the rights and welfare of patients. These entities, known as the Institutional Review Board (IRB) and the Data and Safety Monitoring Board (DSMB), are completely independent from the studies' investigators and sponsors. They have full authority to veto or stop any trial that does not conform to a rigid set of standards. The IRB and DSMB regularly and periodically review all clinical trials to ensure that patients' rights and safety are always protected. These boards have the responsibility to ensure that all clinical trials are both ethically and scientifically sound. Some trials are terminated prematurely because of risk to the participants. Others may be terminated prematurely because their benefits to patients are clear. Premature termination of a clinical trial confirms that the IRB and DSMB are doing exactly what these entities were designed to do.

The clinical trial is the yardstick by which we measure the effectiveness of any new therapy, and it may provide surprising results that defy logic. In learning to live with coronary heart disease, you are likely to hear a lot about clinical trials. You are about to hear about a very important clinical trial involving a drug called cholestyramine and how it changed our understanding of the role of cholesterol.

The Good, the Bad, and the Ugly Facts about Cholesterol

Recall that dietary fat and cholesterol are absorbed by the small intestine and then transported to the liver where they are repackaged as LDL, HDL, and other lipoproteins. If we could somehow prevent the absorption of dietary fat and cholesterol, we might be able lower our cholesterol and LDL levels. Cholestyramine (Questran) is an agent that does just that. To be absorbed by the intestine, cholesterol particles must be emulsified (dissolved) by bile acids. Orally ingested cholestyramine binds to bile acids in the small intestine and prevents the absorption of dietary cholesterol. The cholesterol–bile acid–cholestyramine complex is not absorbed and is eventually excreted in the stool. In the late 1970s, it was not clear whether eliminating cholesterol this way would affect the development of coronary heart disease.

The Lipid Research Clinic Coronary Primary Prevention Trial (LRC-CPPT) was designed to answer that question and others. Published in 1984, this landmark trial was the first study to demonstrate that medical therapy designed to lower cholesterol could save lives. People who were treated with oral cholestyramine for an average of seven years had a 20.3 percent reduction in their LDL cholesterol. This laboratory benefit had a real effect on lives: people taking the drug saw a 19 percent reduction in death and new heart attacks. That's right—there was a 1 percent decline in adverse cardiovascular events for every 1 percent reduction in total cholesterol. This was a revolutionary outcome. Lowering cholesterol saved lives. Cholestyramine users were also less likely to have positive stress tests, suffer from symptomatic angina, or require coronary bypass surgery. The LRC-CPPT was the first prospective clinical trial that produced unequivocal evidence supporting the importance of cholesterol reduction as a means of reducing the risk of coronary heart disease. Lowering cholesterol soon became the goal of every person with coronary heart disease.

While effective, cholestyramine treatment has its problems. Participants in the LRC-CPPT had to take cholestyramine up to six times a day. Severe constipation was a universal complaint. In addition to blocking the absorption of cholesterol, cholestyramine blocks the absorption of many essential vitamins and minerals, and some medications. Patients taking cholestyramine require close monitoring. Not surprisingly, cholestyramine is no longer the treatment of choice for lowering LDL cholesterol. The LRC-CPPT targeted only dietary cholesterol, and dietary fat is only one source of cholesterol. Might we do better by blocking other sources of cholesterol?

In response to bodily demands, the liver makes cholesterol. Because the liver may make more cholesterol than we take in from dietary sources, it would be beneficial if we could regulate the amount of cholesterol that is made in the liver. This is exactly what a group of drugs commonly referred to as statins do. Statins work in the liver

TABLE 4.2 *Commonly Available Statin Agents*

Brand Name	Generic Name
Mevacor	lovastatin
Pravachol	pravastatin
Zocor	simvastatin
Lescol	fluvastatin
Lipitor	atorvastatin
Crestor	rosuvastatin

by interfering in a chemical step in the synthesis of cholesterol. They are the most effective means currently on the market of lowering cholesterol. Table 4.2 lists the commonly available statin agents in the United States.

Statin agents are one of the great medical breakthroughs of the twentieth century. These drugs really work, and their impact on public health has been enormous. On average, statin agents can reduce LDL cholesterol 30 to 50 percent, far more than any other means. More important, this dramatic decline in LDL is associated with a dramatic decline in myocardial infarction and cardiovascular-related death.

Several prospective, randomized, placebo-controlled clinical trials showed that a reduction in cholesterol is associated with a reduction in cardiovascular mortality. In these trials, the statin agents were used in patients without known heart disease (primary prevention) and in patients with a history of prior heart disease (secondary prevention). In every instance, the decline in LDL was dramatic, and in every instance, this decline in LDL was associated with a significant reduction in cardiovascular-associated mortality. This "mortality benefit" associated with statin use occurred whether the drug was used for primary or secondary prevention, in high-risk and in low-risk patients. Collectively, these studies underscore the importance of cholesterol reduction in reducing cardiovascular mortality. This principle has become the cornerstone of the treatment of coronary heart disease.

Many people use the words "cholesterol" and "LDL" interchangeably, even though cholesterol is only one component of the lipoprotein we refer to as LDL. Everyone agrees that LDL contains "bad cholesterol" and that the lower your LDL level, the lower your chance of developing coronary heart disease. High density lipoprotein

(HDL) contains the same cholesterol as LDL does. Why, then, is it called "good cholesterol"?

HDL is a *reverse transport molecule.* The primary function of HDL is to remove cholesterol that is trapped within macrophages and foam cells in the blood vessel wall. HDL repackages this excess cholesterol and returns it to the liver for elimination in bile. It acts like a chemical vacuum cleaner, actually removing cholesterol from atherosclerotic plaque. HDL molecules have been shown to grow in size as they travel through the body, scavenging excess cholesterol. In addition, HDL has been shown to inhibit the adhesion of platelets to vascular endothelium, reduce vascular inflammation, and promote the formation of nitric oxide. In many ways, HDL is an antidote for toxic LDL. There are several different subforms of HDL, but not all of them are equally effective in antagonizing the atherosclerotic process. Unfortunately, measuring all the subforms of HDL is neither a practical nor a cost-effective laboratory test. For now, a composite measurement of all HDL subforms will need to suffice.

A person's risk of developing coronary heart disease is related to the relative amounts of circulating LDL and HDL. Some people have high levels of cholesterol, predominantly LDL, and a great deal of atherosclerosis, while others have an equally high level of cholesterol, with a high HDL, and very little atherosclerosis. Low levels of LDL can cause atherosclerosis if the HDL level is also low. In fact, low *HDL has become just as important a risk factor for the development of coronary heart disease as high LDL.*

It is in your best interest to have an HDL level that is as high as possible. HDL levels can be raised by doing aerobic exercise, maintaining an ideal body weight, committing to a diet that is high in fiber and monosaturated fats, and not smoking. Modest alcohol consumption (one to two drinks per day) has also been shown to produce a small increase in HDL cholesterol, though consuming much more alcohol than this can cause problems related to the alcohol itself. Despite intense efforts in all these areas, some people continue to have low levels of HDL. For them, increasing the level of HDL is very hard to do.

Some drugs help raise HDL levels. Niacin (nicotinic acid, or vitamin B6) seems to be one of the more effective ones, raising HDL levels between 15 and 30 percent. Unfortunately, current preparations of niacin are not practical means of raising HDL and may even be dangerous. Niacin is sometimes used as a dietary supplement in doses of 10 to 20 milligrams per day, but to raise HDL levels, doses of 1,000 to 3,000 milligrams per day are often required. At these doses, the frequency of side effects (facial flushing, sweating, or headaches) is high. For this reason, many people do not like taking niacin. The future possibility of using niacin to raise HDL levels holds some promise. Researchers have identified the mechanism by which niacin causes unpleasant flushing, raising the possibility that these side effects may be blocked by certain medications. Clinical trials will be needed to establish the efficacy of this approach to taking niacin. Because of the possibility of drug interactions, use niacin with caution and only with the advice and supervision of your physician.

Fibrates are another class of drugs that can help raise HDL levels. Gemfibrozil and fenofibrate are the two most commonly used. Fibrates usually raise HDL only 10 to 15 percent. They are much better at lowering triglyceride levels and are generally not used as a first-line means of raising HDL.

Researchers are working intensely to find out how to raise HDL levels. One avenue of research investigates how some constituent HDL particles that return to the liver are actually converted to LDL. This *transfer* of HDL constituents within the liver is facilitated by a special protein called *cholesteryl ester transfer protein* (CETP). The more CETP you have, the less HDL you seem to make and the more atherosclerosis you develop. Wouldn't it be interesting to prevent this internal repackaging of HDL (into LDL) by inhibiting the activity of CETP? Until recently, this was not possible.

CETP inhibitors are a new class of drugs currently under development as a means of reversing the formation of atherosclerosis. In animal studies, inhibiting CETP was associated with a dramatic increase in HDL levels. Torcetrapib is a CETP inhibitor that offered some promise as the first drug that was capable of producing a significant rise in HDL. Several small clinical trials had suggested that patients treated with torcetrapib increased their HDL levels by as much 60 to 100 percent. This was far more than any means currently available. Unfortunately, in 2006 a large clinical trial studying the efficacy of torcetrapib found an increased incidence of death in the group receiving this drug. The study was stopped, and the manufacturer of the drug decided to halt production. Several other CETP inhibitors are currently under development, but many unanswered questions remain. At this point it isn't clear whether HDL elevated by this means will have the same effect on reducing coronary heart disease as HDL elevated by traditional means or whether this elevation will translate to an improvement in mortality. The long-term side effects of using this type of drug are also unknown. Nonetheless, the possibility of using CETP inhibitors to prevent or regress coronary heart disease is an exciting development in the treatment of coronary heart disease.

Altering the relative amounts of circulating LDL and HDL is only one front in the larger battle against coronary heart disease. Remember that while the accumulation of LDL within the blood vessel wall is an important part of the atherosclerotic process, the subsequent inflammatory reaction within the blood vessel wall is equally important. Recognizing this inflammatory process and fighting it are essential to learning to live with coronary heart disease.

Recognizing Vascular Inflammation

Often when you get sick, you get a fever. The fever is a marker for the inflammatory process taking place while you fight the infection. The infection may be located anywhere in the body. A fever doesn't tell you where the infection is, but it suggests that you have one, somewhere. Inflammation of the blood vessels is a similar process but on a smaller scale. Inflammation of the blood vessels does not produce a fever, but your body often reacts with the production of a protein that is indicative of an ongoing inflammatory process. This protein circulates in the blood and, if discovered in a blood test, alerts you to the presence of inflammation.

There are many serum markers of inflammation; for inflammation of the blood vessels, the nonspecific inflammatory marker is the *high-sensitivity C-reactive protein* (hs-CRP). The hs-CRP is the most widely studied tool to identify people with arterial inflammation. An elevated hs-CRP is not specific for arterial inflammation, however, because there are many other possible causes for an elevated hs-CRP besides arterial inflammation. Nonetheless, people with an elevated hs-CRP have a higher risk for cardiovascular events than those whose hs-CRP is normal. In fact, an elevated hs-CRP seems to identify people at risk for adverse cardiovascular events over and above what can be explained by an elevated LDL cholesterol alone. The availability of hs-CRP testing introduces a new dimension to assessing the risk of developing atherosclerosis-related cardiac events.

The usefulness of the hs-CRP in identifying people at risk of a coronary event was first reported in the *New England Journal of Medicine* in 2002. In a prospective review of nearly 28,000 patients, hs-CRP, LDL, and HDL levels were correlated with cardiovascular outcomes over an eight-year period. Low levels of LDL and low levels of hs-CRP were associated with the most favorable prognosis. Not surprisingly, elevated levels of LDL and low levels of hs-CRP were associated with an increase in cardiovascular events. Much to everyone's surprise, *low* levels of LDL and *elevated* hs-CRP were associated with a significant increase in cardiovascular events. Low LDL and elevated hs-CRP indicated a worse prognosis than an elevated LDL did. Patients with a combination of elevated hs-CRP and elevated LDL had the highest incidence of cardiovascular events. Clearly, the presence of arterial inflammation made the cardiovascular prognosis worse. This study suggested that knowledge of the hs-CRP level provides predictive information that is beyond what is conveyed by the LDL level alone. It underscores the important concept that coronary heart disease is caused by the combined effects of cholesterol accumulation and the development of arterial inflammation.

Elevated hs-CRP levels put a person at risk for cardiovascular events, regardless of whether their LDL is elevated or not. There is an ongoing debate about whether an elevated hs-CRP is the chicken or the egg of coronary heart disease. Considerable evidence is accumulating that hs-CRP may be more than a passive marker of inflammation. It may actually be an *active contributor* to the inflammatory atherosclerotic process.

It seems that elevated levels of hs-CRP can fuel the atherosclerotic process. For example, the inflammation that produces high hs-CRP levels alters the lining of the blood vessel, making it stickier and thus easier for circulating LDL molecules and monocytes to adhere to it.

Circulating hs-CRP also seems to enhance the ability of monocytes to penetrate the arterial wall and initiate the plaque-building process. Finally, hs-CRP activates the blood-clotting system, facilitating the formation of blood clots within the coronary artery and promoting the development of an acute coronary syndrome.

Hs-CRP may be the response to some other inflammatory process (possibly an infection) and, once elevated, may ignite the atherosclerotic process culminating in an acute coronary syndrome. There is currently much investigation focusing on the link between an infectious process and triggering of coronary heart disease. There have been no firm conclusions supporting or refuting any link to an infectious trigger to the atherosclerotic process. Either as an active ingredient or as a passive marker of inflammation, hs-CRP is clearly involved in the atherosclerosis story. Measuring your hs-CRP is just as important as measuring your LDL and HDL levels. Doing so involves a simple blood test that is readily available.

Learning to live with coronary heart disease means you will need to be tested for elevated hs-CRP levels, eliminate them, and prevent their reemergence over time—but how? It turns out that aspirin, the well-known fever reducer and anti-inflammatory agent, also works with hs-CRP. Compared to a placebo, aspirin has been shown to reduce the level of hs-CRP, although the degree is rather modest. Aspirin's greatest benefit is linked to its ability to prevent blood clot formation (see chapter 5). As a drug with more than one clinical effect, aspirin is referred to as having pleiotropic (plī´-ə-trō´-pĭk) properties. Other great pleiotropic drugs of our time are the statin agents.

In addition to dramatically lowering LDL, statins reduce the level of hs-CRP, significantly reducing arterial inflammation. Some statins may also produce a mild increase in HDL. In fact, there is growing evidence that statin agents, via their pleiotropic actions, may reduce preexisting atherosclerotic plaque.

In a recent clinical trial entitled REVERSAL, atherosclerotic plaque regression was clearly shown to occur in patients treated with high doses of statin agents. This plaque regression was, in turn, associated with a reduction in clinical cardiovascular events, although these benefits occurred only in patients who experienced a decline in *both* LDL and hs-CRP. The ability to reduce LDL and hs-CRP may be specific to certain statin agents. We are still learning a lot about how and when to use statins (see chapter 6). In addition to reducing LDL and elevating HDL, then, you need to fight inflammation. Medications have come a long way in helping people accomplish all this, but having the right genes helps.

The Right Genes

Everyone knows someone who developed coronary heart disease even though they "did all the right things." Coronary heart disease can affect even people with normal or low LDL. There is great variability in how coronary heart disease evolves. For some of us, coronary heart disease may develop very early in our lives. For others, much later. In some families, coronary heart disease affects multiple members while they are relatively young. In others, longevity is the rule with virtually no instances of symptomatic heart disease. It is difficult to say how large a role family history plays in the development of coronary heart disease. Heart disease in some families may simply represent a focus of environmental factors, such as a tendency toward tobacco use, poor dietary habits, or a sedentary lifestyle. In others, it may be a true reflection of a genetic predisposition for hypertension or diabetes. There is little question, however, that the degree to which we develop and ultimately manifest coronary heart disease is, in part, determined by our genetic makeup.

One of the ways in which this genetic difference is expressed is in how our bodies manufacture lipoproteins. In some people, genetic makeup facilitates the production of LDL, which, in turn, promotes the formation of coronary heart disease. In others, genetics favor the production of HDL, which retards the atherosclerotic process. While LDL and HDL are well-known cholesterol transport envelopes, many other lipoproteins may work with these molecules to either promote or retard the atherosclerotic process. These are considered to be "helper" lipoproteins. Some of them help enhance the favorable actions of HDL. Others help enhance the detrimental actions of LDL. Genetics play a large role in determining in whom and to what extent these lesser known lipoproteins modulate the atherosclerotic process.

Lipoprotein (a), referred to as "Lp little a" or Lp (a), is one such molecule. This interesting lipoprotein has chemical characteristics of both blood-clotting factors and lipids. Acting as a lipid, Lp (a) seems to enhance the actions of circulating LDL, allowing it to damage the endothelial lining, penetrate the arterial wall more easily, and initiate the atherosclerotic process. Acting as a blood-clotting factor, Lp (a) can also promote the formation of blood clots on atherosclerotic plaque. It is no surprise that individuals with higher levels of Lp (a) have a higher incidence of atherosclerotic disease, angina, and myocardial infarctions.

Lipoprotein (a) levels are partially determined by genetic makeup. While equally present in men and women, Lp (a) levels are considerably higher in the African American population. An elevated Lp (a) level is one of the most common lipid abnormalities identified in people with premature atherosclerotic disease. Lp (a) levels may also rise in response to an ongoing medical condition. Many people with diabetes or renal failure have significant elevations in Lp (a) levels, which may in part be responsible for the high incidence of coronary heart disease in individuals with these conditions. There is little question that an elevated Lp (a) level is bad for you. It acts as an accelerant for the formation of atherosclerosis, much like lighter fluid on charcoal. Testing for serum Lp (a) levels is available, but we do not yet know what to do with the information provided by the tests. Lp (a) levels are notoriously resistant to conventional treatment with cholesterol-lowering therapies. For now, measuring LP (a) is not part of the standard assessment of patients with coronary heart disease.

Not all genetically determined lipoproteins are bad, as is made clear by the residents of Limone sul Garda, a small town outside Milan, Italy. These fortunate people have an extraordinarily low incidence of atherosclerotic disease. Extensive study of the residents of this town has confirmed that many of them have a unique lipoprotein that protects them against the development of coronary heart disease. *Apolipoprotein A-I* (apo A-I) is a lipoprotein that everyone has. In fact, it is a major component of HDL. In the residents of Limone sul Garda, this lipoprotein is slightly different. While their levels of HDL are not very high, they seem to have a super efficient means of combating coronary heart disease. The residents of Limone sul Garda appear to have a gene that has altered the structure of apo A-I to their benefit. Now referred to as apo A-I Milano, this lipoprotein enhances the protective aspects of HDL. Apo A-I Milano is a very exciting molecule. By enhancing the actions of HDL, apo A-I Milano actually helps remove cholesterol from atherosclerotic plaque.

"Where can I get some apo A-I Milano?" you might ask. Until recently, if you didn't happen to be related to natives of Limone sul Garda, you were out of luck, but now apo A-I Milano can be prepared in the laboratory by recombinant DNA technology. A study giving intravenous apo A-I Milano to people with preexisting coronary heart disease showed, to everyone's amazement, that it seemed to work. A five-week infusion of apo A-I Milano was associated with a significant decrease in the size of atherosclerotic plaque in individuals with coronary heart disease. The short- and long-term prognosis for people treated with this agent is not clear. Nor are the short- and long-term side effects of prolonged use of this new compound known. Nonetheless, the prospect of retarding or reversing coronary heart disease with a drug infusion is exciting.

Genetic variations in the nature of coronary heart disease involve more than variations in the quantity and quality of circulating lipoproteins. Men and women tend to develop and express coronary heart disease very differently: men tend to develop coronary heart disease at a younger age. After menopause, however, women tend to acquire coronary heart disease rapidly, catching up with men and eventually exceeding them with respect to its severity and ultimately mortality. Coronary heart disease in women may be different than it is in men. The reason for this difference in the development of coronary heart disease has been the subject of much debate. The most likely explanation is that in premenopausal women, circulating reproductive hormones may somehow retard coronary heart disease.

Estrogen, the Double-Edged Sword of Coronary Heart Disease

Estrogen and progesterone are the principal female reproductive hormones. Variations in the levels of these hormones produce a woman's ovulation cycle and help stimulate the breasts and uterus in anticipation of conception. Estrogen and progesterone also have important effects on nonreproductive organs, including the heart, liver, and skeletal system. The effects of estrogen have been more extensively studied than the effects of progesterone.

Estrogen exerts its effects on the cardiovascular system through various direct and indirect mechanisms. Acting directly, estrogen molecules are able to enter cardiac muscle cells and the endothelial cells lining blood vessel walls. As we saw in chapter 2, when the heart requires more blood to meet its energy demands, the coronary arteries automatically enlarge. Estrogen enhances this autoregulatory process. In addition, circulating estrogen may offer some protection against developing coronary heart disease. Estrogen reduces the tendency for oxidized LDL molecules to penetrate the blood vessel wall and initiate the formation of atherosclerotic plaques. Thus, in normal arteries, estrogen seems to have the beneficial effects of enhancing the arteries' normally adaptive function as well as making them more resistant to the formation of atherosclerotic plaque. The key to these important observations is that the processes occur in *normal* arteries. Once atherosclerosis is established, these favorable actions of estrogen may not be so apparent. Recognizing that the action of estrogen depends on whether the arteries are normal or not is important in understanding the role that *hormone replacement therapy* (HRT) may play in women following menopause.

Estrogen has many indirect actions that seem to be as important as (or even more important than) the direct ones. Estrogen can alter cholesterol metabolism. It can decrease the amount of circulating LDL and simultaneously raise the amount of beneficial HDL in the blood. The low incidence of coronary heart disease in premenopausal women may be related to this favorable alteration in the relative amounts of LDL and HDL. This observation has led to the inference that replacing these hormones after menopause may offer women some protection against the development of coronary heart disease. This conclusion, however, may not necessarily be warranted, for HRT may have both beneficial and harmful effects.

The female reproductive system is exquisitely sensitive to the levels of circulating estrogen and progesterone. Accordingly, the body tightly controls the amount of estrogen and progesterone it makes. Through a complex method of monitoring and synthesis, the body makes only as much of each hormone as is needed. Administering these hormones by pill or by cutaneous patch is nowhere near as well controlled as the body's own processes. There is legitimate concern that hormone replacement will overstimulate the breast tissue and uterus and may predispose some women to cancer. Estrogen also has the unwanted effect of activating the coagulation system and, in doing so, favoring the formation of blood clots. This tendency of estrogen to stimulate blood clot formation may more than offset the benefit of inhibiting atherosclerotic plaque formation. Women receiving supplemental estrogen have an increased incidence of blood clots forming in various locations. Blood clots can form in the leg veins, leading to a condition referred to as *thrombophlebitis* (thräm´-bō-fli-bī´-təs). The blood clot may remain in the leg vein, causing pain and swelling, or it may break off and migrate to the lungs. This life-threatening disruption of the blood supply to the lungs is referred to as a *pulmonary embolus.*

In the heart, this tendency to form clots can have equally dire consequences. Estrogen can facilitate clot formation within the heart's chambers or on one of the valves. If this clot dislodges, it can travel through the arteries, leading to a stroke or disruption of the blood supply to some other vital organ. A blood clot can form on the wall of just about any vessel. The small caliber of the coronary arteries makes them particularly vulnerable to clot formation. Because clot formation at the site of an inflamed atherosclerotic plaque is an essential ingredient for a heart attack, by increasing the risk of forming a clot in a coronary artery, HRT might increase a woman's risk of having a heart attack. While the likelihood of any of these occurrences is small, HRT (especially for women who smoke) clearly increases the risk of blood clot formation and its subsequent complications. So there is a dilemma with hormone replacement.

Randomized clinical research trials are essential in evaluating any new form of therapy. Two prospective, randomized, double-blind, placebo-controlled trials in the 1990s have evaluated HRT for the prevention of coronary heart disease. They are the Women's Health Initiative (WHI), which began in the 1990s and involved 16,608 women, and

Heart and Estrogen/Progestin Replacement Study (HERS), involving 2,763 women.

The WHI was a *primary prevention* trial. It was designed to see whether HRT could prevent the development of coronary heart disease after menopause. The WHI was stopped prematurely when the DSMB noticed a trend toward an increase in the incidence of breast cancer without an apparent cardiovascular benefit in women taking HRT. Critics of the WHI suggest that the trial was poorly designed, because hormone replacement was started too late after menopause. The average age of patients in the WHI was 63 years old, and therefore it is likely that in some of these women, the atherosclerotic process had begun long before the initiation of treatment. Thus it might be difficult to see any cardiovascular benefit in patients treated with hormone replacement. While this may be a valid criticism of the trial, the WHI certainly underscored the potential dangers of HRT, documenting an increased incidence of stroke, pulmonary blood clots, and breast cancer in patients treated with hormone replacement.

The HERS trial was a similar trial examining the role of estrogen replacement in women. It was designed as a *secondary prevention* trial. It evaluated the value of hormone replacement in women with preexisting atherosclerotic disease. In this trial, after four years, there was no significant difference in the frequency of cardiovascular events between the women taking hormone replacement and the women taking placebo.

Based on these randomized trials, hormone replacement for the prevention of atherosclerotic disease is no longer recommended. There are, however, many unanswered questions. Should different hormones be tried? If so, at what dose and how should they be delivered? Would the results have been different had treatment begun either before or immediately after the start of menopause? There are several prospective studies under way to address these and other important questions. You will hear more about hormone replacement therapy in the years to come. For now, HRT is not indicated as a means of preventing coronary heart disease in women following menopause. Depending on your particular health, your doctor may choose to use hormone supplementation to treat other medical conditions.

Variations in hormone levels influence the relationship between

LDL, HDL, and the blood-clotting system. Certain medical conditions can do that and more. Diabetes is one of these.

Diabetes and Coronary Heart Disease

Everything we do requires energy. Our muscles require energy to help us move. Our kidneys require energy to filter blood. Our brains require energy to let us think. Every cell in our body requires energy to enable it to perform its specific function. Glucose is the principal fuel that our cells use to manufacture that energy. Insulin facilitates the entry of glucose into the cells. In effect, it is the key that unlocks the door to energy factories. Without insulin, our cells cannot effectively manufacture the energy we need. *Diabetes* (properly called *diabetes mellitus*) is a term that encompasses various disorders characterized by an inability to use glucose effectively. But diabetes involves much more than glucose metabolism. The inability to use glucose effectively as a source of energy is the first serious biochemical alteration of what soon becomes a cascade of such alterations. The byproducts of this altered metabolism damage nearly every organ in the body. Much, but not all, of the organ damage inflicted by diabetes is a direct result of the atherosclerotic plaque that blossoms in the large and small arteries. Diabetes mellitus significantly magnifies all the problems of coronary heart disease.

There are two principal types of diabetes. Type I diabetes is a result of autoimmune destruction of the cells in the pancreas that produce insulin. The body inadvertently creates antibodies that target and destroy the insulin-producing pancreatic beta cells. In genetically predisposed individuals, this cellular destruction may begin at an early age, leading to insufficient insulin production and elevated glucose levels in childhood or adolescence. Type II diabetes is a disease of adults and is sometimes referred to as *maturity onset diabetes*. It is much more common than type I and is the result of several interrelated developments. In genetically predisposed individuals, aging results in a decreased sensitivity to the insulin the pancreas makes, creating the high glucose levels that characterize diabetes. Given the inability to use the high levels of glucose effectively, the body seeks alternative forms of energy, breaking down excess body fat into usable fuels known as *fatty acids*. In the liver, these free fatty acids are converted to excess triglycerides and LDL. People with diabetes characteristically have high levels of triglycerides and LDL.

The LDL of people with diabetes is also different and more prone to form coronary heart disease. People with diabetes have small and densely packed LDL particles that seem to be particularly effective in penetrating the endothelial lining of a blood vessel, activating macrophages and initiating coronary heart disease. The creation of these abnormal LDL particles is driven by a complex interaction between the abnormally high triglyceride level and the low HDL level that many people with diabetes have. Unable to use glucose efficiently, people with diabetes rely on free fatty acids for energy. Triglycerides are a byproduct of the increased free fatty acid metabolism. In someone with high triglycerides, the cholesteryl ester transfer protein (CETP) works overtime, depleting stores of HDL and converting triglycerides to small and very dense LDL particles. The result is the emergence of high levels of a very atherogenic LDL accompanied by low levels of HDL. This combination is likely to lead to coronary heart disease. In people with diabetes, the battle against coronary heart disease must be waged on three fronts: lowering LDL, raising HDL, and minimizing fasting triglycerides. That is why people with diabetes are frequently prescribed a fibrate or another triglyceride-lowering agent *in addition to a statin*.

The link between diabetes and heart disease involves more than aggressive atherosclerotic plaque formation. Sensing the elevated glucose levels, the body actually tries to produce more of the resistant insulin. The markedly elevated insulin levels, while inefficient in lowering the glucose, are very efficient in activating the blood-clotting system and stimulating the inflammatory process that characterizes coronary heart disease. Diabetes, by favoring the formation of a highly abnormal lipid profile, activating the blood-clotting system, and stimulating an inflammatory response thus creates a perfect storm for the formation of coronary heart disease and all its complications.

How diabetes promotes these abnormalities is not entirely clear. Current research is focusing on the role of a hormone called *adiponectin*. Adiponectin is produced by fat cells and is secreted into the bloodstream. All of us make adiponectin. Elevated adiponectin levels improve sensitivity to insulin, reduce tissue inflammation, lower LDL, and even raise HDL. Low adiponectin levels produce the opposite effects and are associated with type II diabetes.

Something happens when obesity sets in to reduce the normal production of adiponectin. Could type II diabetes be a condition of abnormally low adiponectin production? Perhaps. If there were a way to raise adiponectin levels, we might be able to block many of the adverse effects of diabetes. When administered to animals with diabetes, adiponectin seems to prevent the expected adverse risk factor profile and may even prevent the formation of coronary heart disease. Human trials to illuminate the link between adiponectin and diabetes are still in their early stages and are not yet conclusive. For now, people with diabetes must aggressively manage glucose and cholesterol levels and take medications to prevent and treat vascular disease. These are the mainstays of diabetic therapy.

If you walk on fresh snow, you leave footprints that remain until the snow melts or new snow falls. The footprints record your presence long after you are gone. Similarly, if your blood glucose becomes elevated for a period, your red blood cells adapt to the higher glucose levels by producing a protein called *glycosylated hemoglobin* (hemoglobin A1c). If your glucose levels are persistently low, your red blood cells make less hemoglobin A1c. Thus, the hemoglobin A1c level, like footprints in the snow, is indicative of where your blood glucose level has been over an extended time. Hemoglobin A1c levels are measured for a three-month period. An elevated hemoglobin A1c is indicative of persistent poor glucose control and is associated with a higher risk for diabetic complications. Conversely, a reduced hemoglobin A1c is indicative of good glucose control and is associated with a favorable prognosis.

People with diabetes need to pay close attention to their hemoglobin A1c. There are excellent data to show that a reduction of just 1 percent in hemoglobin A1c (such as 8.5 percent decreasing to 7.5 percent) causes a 35 percent reduction in the incidence of microvascular complications involving small vessels of the eyes, kidneys, and feet. The usual goal for hemoglobin A1c is less than 7 percent, which generally means fasting blood glucose of less than 120 mg/dl (milligrams per deciliter) and less than 140 mg/dl two hours after meals. These are not easy goals to achieve, but the subsequent improvement in prognosis is well worth the effort. If you have diabetes, it is essential for you to achieve very tight control of your glucose levels. As noted, much of the benefit derived by tight glucose management involves the prevention of microvascular complications; it is less clear whether tight glucose control affects complications related to large vessel atherosclerosis, including the vessels supplying the brain, heart, and aorta. Prevention of this large vessel atherosclerosis seems more dependent on cholesterol management than on glucose management.

There is little question that individuals with either type I or type II diabetes have a markedly increased incidence of heart attacks and stroke. In fact, an individual with diabetes has a risk of having a heart attack that is equal to that of a nondiabetic person who has already had one. Diabetes is *risk equivalent* to having preexisting coronary heart disease. Much of this excess risk can be eliminated by treatment with statin agents. Accordingly, the current standard of care states that every person with diabetes, *regardless* of their cholesterol level, be treated with a statin agent.

Unfortunately, there is not much you can do to avoid type I diabetes if you are genetically predisposed. But the very best way to manage type II diabetes is not to get it. There are many things you can do to prevent or delay your chances of getting type II diabetes. Recognizing whether you are at risk to develop type II diabetes is an important first step. A family history of type I diabetes clearly increases your chances of developing the disease. It is possible to identify people who are prone to diabetes long before they have symptoms or evidence of organ damage. They may exhibit abnormal fasting levels of glucose or have a lipid profile and body build that is typical for future diabetes. This so-called prediabetic condition is sometimes referred to as the *metabolic syndrome*.

Both men and women who have fat stores in their belly and chest (a condition called *truncal obesity*) are more likely to develop metabolic syndrome. Truncal obesity is usually defined as a waist circumference larger than forty inches in men and thirty-five inches in women. Metabolic syndrome can be identified through routine blood testing. The fasting glucose level is somewhat elevated (greater than

100 to 120 mg/dl), triglycerides are elevated, and HDL cholesterol is abnormally low. The LDL level is not necessarily high, but the nature of the LDL in people with metabolic syndrome is highly abnormal. It is the same as the highly atherogenic, small, dense LDL we discussed earlier. There is little question that left untreated, metabolic syndrome increases the risk for cardiovascular disease and diabetes.

In the prediabetic state, lifestyle modifications can play a major role in reducing the chance of developing diabetes. In the 2001 Finnish Diabetes Prevention Study, 522 overweight patients were randomized to receive either intensive counseling for lifestyle modifications or routine care. Lifestyle modifications included a closely monitored diet with reduced saturated fats and increased amounts of fiber, with emphasis on weight reduction and increased physical activity. The results of this study were striking. Over a six-year period, patients who engaged in lifestyle modification activities (the intervention group) reduced their chance of developing diabetes by 58 percent. Aside from a significant reduction in weight, lifestyle modifiers enjoyed the benefit of lower cholesterol levels and lower blood pressure. While not yet documented, the potential impact on the incidence of coronary heart disease and cardiovascular mortality in this group should be enormous. The bottom line: *Don't accept obesity and diabetes as an inevitable sequence of events.* The Finnish Diabetes Prevention Study is just one of many examples of how you can intervene in your own life, take better care of yourself, and improve your health.

Obesity increases a person's chances of developing diabetes, and it also significantly increases a person's risk of developing hypertension. No discussion of coronary heart disease would be complete without considering the role of hypertension.

How Hypertension Hurts

Hypertension (high blood pressure) is usually defined as a systolic blood pressure greater than 140 mm Hg, or a diastolic blood pressure greater than 90 mm Hg. At the very minimum, hypertension inflicts its damage by promoting premature wear and tear of the blood vessels and the heart. To adapt to a higher blood pressure, arteries enlarge and overdevelop their muscular layer. Likewise, the heart tends to enlarge and its walls thicken. This initially adaptive mechanism can progress and cause problems later on. The thick muscular arteries become stiff, no longer responding very well to physiological stimuli. The higher intravascular blood pressure promotes damage to the endothelial lining of the arteries. Collectively, these consequences of hypertension set the stage for the development of atherosclerotic plaque. Hypertension also may contribute to coronary heart disease in ways that are not primarily related to the high blood pressure, because some people are predisposed to developing coronary heart disease due to a chemical mediator that is frequently elevated in people with hypertension.

There are many causes of hypertension. In many instances, the cause is an abnormally high level of a substance called *angiotensin II*. All of us make angiotensin II. It constricts blood vessels and in doing so causes hypertension. Angiotensin II may have effects other than vasoconstriction. At persistently elevated levels, it can wreak havoc inside the body by promoting the abnormal growth of smooth muscle cells, enhancing the inflammatory process, and stimulating fibrosis, the development of scar tissue, and salt retention. (How angiotensin II does this is reviewed in chapter 6 in a discussion of drug treatment for coronary heart disease.)

It's easy to see why avoiding diabetes and hypertension can help you avoid coronary heart disease. If you develop diabetes and hypertension, then the next best thing is to tightly control glucose levels and blood pressure levels by modifying your diet and exercise routine and by taking medications; it is very important to keep these promoters of coronary heart disease in check. You can work at staying thin; you can choose to stay in shape; and you can choose not to smoke.

Choosing Not to Smoke

In the battle against coronary heart disease, some things are beyond your control. Smoking is not one of them. Smokers choose to start smoking and continue to do so despite knowing it is bad for their health. Inhaling cigarette smoke is just about the worst thing you can do to your heart and blood vessels. The inhaled smoke immediately reduces the oxygen content of your blood. The reduced oxygen content of the blood causes the coronary arteries to constrict, limiting the flow of blood to your heart muscle. At the very minimum, smokers' hearts have to work harder on every beat.

Over time, inhaled cigarette smoke induces many changes in the body's regulatory system. Circulating LDL goes up. HDL levels fall. The blood-clotting system is activated, and the body produces numerous inflammatory substances that promote damage to the endothelial lining of the arteries. Does this sound like the familiar recipe for the formation of coronary heart disease? You bet it does. Smokers have over twice the incidence of coronary heart disease and twice the cardiovascular mortality as nonsmokers.

When You Have Multiple Risk Factors

Not many people have only one cardiovascular risk factor. Smokers, for example, tend to have other cardiovascular risk factors, such as high lipids. People who are obese also usually have multiple risk factors. The relative increase in cardiovascular risk brought on by the presence of additional risk factors is not additive, it's *multiplied* (see figure 4.1).

For any single cardiac risk factor you have, the odds of your having a heart attack are two to three times greater than for a person with no risk factors. When a person has multiple risk factors, the odds of having a heart attack skyrocket. If you have multiple risk factors *and* you are obese, you have a very high risk of a heart attack. Fighting the battle of obesity is one of the most important things you can do in the war against coronary heart disease.

Chances are that you weigh a little more than you should. Many people do. There may be some truth to the notion that some people have a large frame or lots of muscle, but we do not have to rely on these old notions because we have objective criteria for defining ideal body weight. This is the body mass index, or BMI. The BMI is nothing more than the ratio of your weight in kilograms to the square

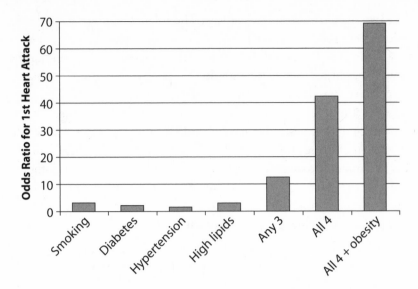

FIGURE 4.1. Impact of multiple risk factors on risk of cardiovascular disease. The presence of any cardiovascular risk factors increases the chances of having a heart attack. Having more than one cardiovascular risk factor increases this risk. Having multiple cardiovascular risk factors multiplies the risk of having a heart attack. Obesity most dramatically compounds heart attack risk. (Adapted from S. Yusuf et al., "Effect of Potentially Modifiable Risk Factors Associated with Myocardial Infarction in 52 Countries [the INTERHEART Study]: Case-Control Study," *Lancet* 364 (2004): 937–52.)

of your height in meters. Several easy-to-use web sites will calculate your BMI for you, such as the American Heart Association site or the National Heart Blood and Lung Institute, part of the National Institutes of Health. A normal BMI is less than 25. A person with a BMI greater than 25 is overweight. Obesity is defined as a BMI of 30 or higher. Using these definitions, almost 60 percent of Americans are considered overweight, and 15 percent of the population is considered obese. Obesity is a serious problem in the United States. It is present and increasing in every age and ethnic group. Obesity tends to start in childhood, and the percentage of obese people under age 65 rises each year. The percentage declines in people over age 65 because of the high mortality rate associated with obesity. The prevalence of obesity is increasing in every city and every state. In many ways, it poses one of the great public health challenges of the twenty-first century.

Most people who develop coronary heart disease wonder whether they did something to cause the disease. As we have seen, in some cases, unfortunately, the answer is probably yes. In others, the answer is not so clear. Some people, seemingly through benign neglect, increase their risk of developing coronary heart disease. Other people actively participate in increasing this risk by engaging in activities that are well known to cause coronary heart disease. For others, coronary heart disease is a product of the genetic cards they were dealt long ago. In any case, there is much you can do to reduce your chance of developing coronary heart disease. In this chapter, we have touched on some of the things you can do to protect your health. As a cardiologist, I encourage you—I *entreat* you—to learn more about diet and exercise and other lifestyle factors, and to take an active role in your current and future health.

FIVE

How Do I Know If I Have Coronary Heart Disease?

....

M any people, and especially any person who has had a heart attack, wonder whether they have coronary heart disease. The symptoms of coronary heart disease can be difficult to recognize, and these symptoms are frequently attributed to something other than the heart (recall James's indigestion from chapter 1). Many people rationalize away their symptoms; that is not a good thing to do. The purpose of this chapter is to describe the symptoms of coronary heart disease and the diagnostic tests that are done to confirm the disease. Everyone should learn to recognize these symptoms because *prompt diagnosis and treatment can be life saving.*

In chapter 3 we saw that atherosclerosis usually reveals itself by producing myocardial ischemia. Strictly speaking, ischemia is a chemical imbalance. It is a metabolic condition that exists when the heart's demand for oxygen exceeds the supply that is delivered by the coronary arteries. It's a lot like hunger, where your need for food exceeds the immediate supply. Atherosclerosis plays a pivotal role in creating an environment that allows this supply-demand imbalance to occur. Atherosclerosis not only narrows the coronary arteries, it also impairs the ability of these arteries to dilate in response to increased metabolic demands. Thus it is useful to think of atherosclerosis as producing two distinct problems in the coronary arteries. One is related to the obstructive effects of atherosclerotic plaque. The other is more subtle and is related to the diseased artery's inability to regulate its size.

In situations when the heart requires more oxygen, such as with exercise, the obstructive nature of atherosclerosis prohibits the coronary arteries from increasing their flow. The mismatch between oxygen

56

supply (as limited by the atherosclerotic coronary arteries) and oxygen demand (as required by the exercising heart) results in a metabolic imbalance. Extending the concept of metabolic imbalance further, we see that myocardial ischemia can also occur when there is an excessive reduction in blood flow without any appreciable increase in oxygen demand. Coronary blood flow can temporarily fall if the diameter of the vessel decreases due to spasm of the blood vessel walls. A small coronary artery spasm superimposed on a small obstructive plaque can suddenly produce a dramatic reduction in coronary blood flow. Once again, the result is myocardial ischemia, but the mechanism is quite different. In this case, the heart's oxygen supply has declined in the setting of normal oxygen demand.

Atherosclerotic coronary arteries may be prone to spasm because of the damage to the endothelial lining and blood vessel wall. Thus, the increased risk of myocardial ischemia is actually the result of both the degree of fixed coronary obstruction (due to plaque) and variable coronary obstruction (due to spasm). People with mostly fixed coronary obstructions tend to develop symptoms of myocardial ischemia in a stable and predictable pattern. They develop ischemia because the increased myocardial oxygen demand (associated with an increased level of physical activity) cannot be met by a similar increase in myocardial blood supply. This pattern of exercise-induced ischemia is referred to as *chronic stable angina pectoris.*

In contrast, other people develop ischemia in a much more variable pattern. Symptoms can come with minimal activity or even at rest. Here the myocardial ischemia is a result of a primary reduction in myocardial blood supply. This pattern of varying degrees of symptoms at rest is sometimes referred to as *unstable angina pectoris,* or *crescendo angina.* Whether the angina symptoms are stable or unstable, they represent a call for help that the person experiencing them must recognize and act on.

Angina Pectoris

Angina pectoris is the heart's call for help. It is the discomfort in the chest (*pectoris*) that frequently accompanies myocardial ischemia.

Notice that I use the word "discomfort" and not the word "pain." The discomfort of myocardial ischemia is rather peculiar and difficult to describe. Some people use the words "pressure" or "tightness," and others use the words "squeezing" or "heaviness," to describe it. For some, no words will do, and they may reflexively motion with a clenched fist across their chest, in a gesture called Levine's sign (the sign is named after the distinguished Harvard cardiologist Samuel Levine, who first noted patients using the clenched fist across their chest as they described their myocardial discomfort).

Strictly speaking, the term *angina pectoris* refers to discomfort that is localized to the chest. The discomfort of myocardial ischemia can be *referred to* (sent to or sensed in) a location other than the chest, but many people use the simpler term *angina* to describe their symptoms. The peculiar sensation of myocardial discomfort can develop in either the arm or the wrist, and may be felt in the shoulder or back. Thus, symptoms can be easily confused with a pulled muscle or arthritis. The sensation of discomfort may also be felt in the neck and extend to the teeth. Symptoms of myocardial discomfort can appear to start in the belly and, as in the case of our patient James, masquerade as indigestion.

Angina has many disguises. But the symptoms of angina can sometimes be recognized because they occur with a certain type of activity. An important distinguishing feature of angina is that it generally occurs with exercise and is relieved by rest. It is more likely to occur with activity after a large meal. Angina is also more likely to occur in the early morning. The intensity and duration of symptoms vary. In some circumstances, the degree of discomfort is overshadowed by other symptoms, such as sweating, shortness of breath, or nausea. It is important to remember that *any repeated or unexplained symptoms require further medical investigation.* You should always be concerned about symptoms that are produced by exercise.

It is difficult to recognize angina. A major reason for the difficulty is that different people experience angina very differently. All of us have varying degrees of tolerance for discomfort; some people are not as bothered by pain as other people. In addition, there may be variation due to gender. Women tend to show considerably more variability in their qualitative descriptions of angina than do men. They may experience more symptoms referred to locations outside the chest. The symptoms may occur more frequently at night. Their symptoms of angina are sometimes described as being "atypical" (although using men as the basis for defining "typical" symptoms is a style of reference that medicine is trying to move away from). Recognizing angina in women can be difficult, and anginal symptoms in women are sometimes misinterpreted or even ignored by both patients and physicians. This variability of anginal symptoms may partly explain why there often seems to be a delay in diagnosing coronary heart disease in women. It may also partly explain why women tend to have fewer diagnostic tests performed than men do. Unfortunately, this delay in recognition and diagnosis of atherosclerotic disease in women may translate to a higher mortality rate. If you are a woman with unexplained or repeated symptoms, you should discuss these symptoms with your doctor before attributing them to something other than your heart.

People with diabetes also may report atypical symptoms of angina. They have what has been referred to as "defective warning systems." Diabetes can damage the nerves that detect sensation, producing a condition called *diabetic neuropathy*. Diabetic neuropathy may extend to the nerves that detect sensation in and around the chest, impairing the person's ability to detect myocardial ischemia. Their sensation of angina can be quite mild. In fact, people with diabetes may not experience angina discomfort at all, and their symptoms may arise solely as a decline in cardiac contracting function. Thus, a person with diabetes may experience only unexplained shortness of breath or fluid retention as a symptom of coronary heart disease. If you are a person with diabetes, you should take these symptoms as seriously as you would take any symptoms of discomfort.

Given the range of symptoms, it can be very difficult to determine whether a person's symptoms are due to angina or whether they are just aches and pains common to all of us. This is obviously a very important determination to make. The earlier angina is recognized, the sooner it can be diagnosed and the underlying coronary heart disease can be treated. Untreated, recurrent angina can progress into a heart attack. Earlier treatment unquestionably improves the prognosis. While the clinical diagnosis of coronary heart disease can be difficult, several types of diagnostic tests are helpful.

It is neither practical nor cost effective to order diagnostic testing for every patient for every type of complaint. All of us have had chest discomfort or vague aches and pains at one time or another. How does your doctor decide who to refer for further testing and who to simply reassure? The answer to this important question lies in considering the symptoms in the context of how likely it is that you have underlying coronary heart disease, based on whether the atherosclerotic risk factor profile places you in a high-risk or low-risk category. This consideration of the probability of having atherosclerosis is referred to as a *Bayesian analysis*. It is the foundation on which physicians decide who to refer for further testing for coronary heart disease.

Does a person's complaints of chest discomfort and neck aches possibly represent angina or not? What conclusion would you draw if the patient was a nonsmoking 25-year-old female with a normal LDL and HDL? Would your interpretation of the symptoms be different if the patient were a 60-year-old male with high blood pressure who has been smoking for forty years and has a very low HDL? While the description of symptoms may be very much the same, the *likelihood* of coronary disease in each of these patients is very different. Based on available statistics, a 60-year-old male with that risk factor profile is at least thirty to forty times more likely to have atherosclerosis than the younger female. Accordingly, his symptoms are far more likely (though not positively) to be related to angina. Additional diagnostic testing in this high-probability group would be more likely to yield clinically useful data. This reliance on assessing the pretest probability of a patient having atherosclerosis should not be interpreted to mean that diagnostic testing does not have a role in individuals with a low probability of having atherosclerosis. This is where clinical judgment and experience come in. There may be all sorts of reasons to pursue diagnostic testing for coronary heart disease, and these decisions are best left up to your physician. Many tests can assist him or her in that determination. Each test has its own set of advantages and disadvantages.

Wouldn't it be great if we could just look inside the heart for atherosclerosis? Unfortunately, imaging the heart, and in particular the coronary arteries, is not a simple matter. The coronary arteries, after all, are quite small, ranging from one to four millimeters in diameter. These tiny blood vessels run through a muscle that is beating sixty to ninety times per minute. This moving target is located in the center of your chest, surrounded by the lungs, breast, and varying amounts of muscle and fat. The ability to image and examine these vessels for the presence or absence of a few millimeters of atherosclerosis is a true technical marvel. X-rays have been the time-honored way of looking inside the body since their discovery by William Roentgen in 1895. At one time or another, virtually all of us have had some kind of x-ray examination. While a simple chest x-ray can see what is inside the chest, it cannot overcome the obstacles of size and motion to visualize the coronary arteries. For this application, computer-enhanced x-rays hold some promise.

Computerized Tomographic Scanning

Computerized tomographic scanning, commonly referred to as CT scanning, has been available for many years. It has been used primarily to image motionless organs like the brain or lung. (If you've ever had a chest x-ray, you'll recall that you were asked to hold your breath while the x-ray was taken, to stop the motion of the lungs.) Accurately imaging a small and beating heart is far more challenging. With the aid of a computer, multiple x-ray beams are projected at the heart from many different directions. The multiple x-ray images are taken in a precisely timed manner. These images are then reassembled by computer and digitally enhanced. The resulting circumferential image of the heart is like viewing the heart in slices; it is often referred to as a *tomogram.*

To get an accurate representation of the cardiac anatomy, multiple thin x-ray slices of the heart must be obtained. The current standard for cardiac images is sixty-four separate slices, though scanners now in development may be able to acquire considerably more. To negate the effect of cardiac motion, the images are recorded in fractions of a second. These rapidly acquired and computer-enhanced CT scanners are commonly referred to as *ultrafast* CT scanners, or *electron beam tomographic* (EBT) scanners. They have become increasingly popular as a means of screening for coronary heart disease.

Ultrafast CT scans can provide images of the coronary arteries, but the current resolution of the images (that is, the ability to see fine details) is insufficient to make accurate determinations about the size and nature of the atherosclerotic plaque. Ultrafast CT scans are very good at determining whether there is any calcium in the coronary artery wall. Figure 5.1 depicts normal and abnormal cross-sectional views of the heart obtained from an ultrafast CT scan.

Atherosclerotic plaque frequently contains some calcium, which is a byproduct of the inflammatory process that produces atherosclerosis. More calcium in the blood vessel wall implies that more atherosclerosis is present. The amount of calcium present is reflected in a calcium score that is calculated for the heart, which correlates with the extent of coronary atherosclerosis. Ultrafast CT scans can detect coronary heart disease in about 90 percent of cases when the calcium score is used.

Although ultrafast CT scanning exposes the patient to more radiation than a simple chest x-ray, it is entirely noninvasive and a very safe way of detecting coronary atherosclerosis. Unfortunately, it does have several drawbacks. It is not 100 percent sensitive for detecting atherosclerosis because not all atherosclerotic plaque is calcified. Some patients have coronary atherosclerosis but do not have much calcium in the blood vessel wall. Either they do not have a positive ultrafast CT scan or they have a positive scan that underestimates the severity of the atherosclerotic disease. This may be particularly true in younger people.

In patients with clearly positive studies, additional important information is often lacking. For example, some patients, particularly older patients, may have a substantial amount of calcium deposited in the coronary artery wall yet have little obstruction of coronary blood flow. An ultrafast CT scan, while accurately suggesting that atherosclerosis may be present, does not provide any information on the severity of the obstruction produced by atherosclerotic plaque.

For these reasons, a significantly positive ultrafast CT scan usually requires additional diagnostic testing, and because of its limitations, ultrafast CT scanning has not been universally embraced by the medical community as a useful tool for the diagnosis of coronary heart disease. The technology of ultrafast CT scanners is rapidly evolving,

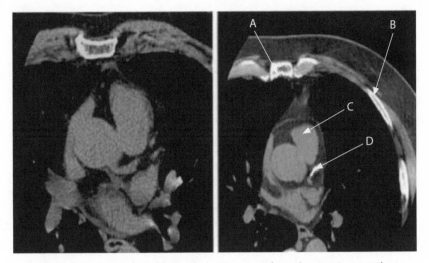

FIGURE 5.1. One frame each of ultrafast CT scans of two hearts. A normal heart is shown on the left, and an abnormal heart is shown on the right: (A) breastbone; (B) rib; (C) pulmonary artery; (D) calcium in coronary artery. This type of image can clearly document the presence of atherosclerosis, but it does not provide accurate information about the degree to which an artery is narrowed. (From www.radiologyinfo.org/en/info.cfm?pg=ct_calscoring.)

however. With additional development, it is possible that in the future, ultrafast CT scanning may be able to provide important information about the nature of the atherosclerotic plaque and how likely it is to rupture and produce a myocardial infarction. For now, ultrafast CT scanning is primarily a screening tool that provides limited anatomical information.

Having anatomical information about the heart is good, but it is usually not good enough. When evaluating coronary heart disease, considering only the anatomical information is like opening the hood of a used car and saying, "Nice engine. It looks pretty good." What you really want to know is how the car drives. You want a functional assessment of the engine. The same holds true for the heart. Doctors want a functional assessment of the impact of any coronary disease. A stress test provides that functional assessment of your "engine" and is one of the most common ways to evaluate coronary heart disease.

A stress test typically does exactly what it says. It stresses the heart, albeit in a controlled manner, to see if myocardial ischemia can be provoked. If it can be, then there must be a functionally significant atherosclerotic obstruction of the coronary arteries . . . *somewhere.* A stress test is not very good at telling us the location of a coronary obstruction. It does not provide the same type of anatomical information that an ultrafast CT scan does. It does, however, provide useful insights regarding your heart's response to stress and, with these insights, important information about the likelihood of future cardiovascular events. A stress test is the most commonly employed diagnostic test to detect and assess the severity of coronary heart disease. There are many ways to stress the heart. The most common way is for the patient to walk on a treadmill under close supervision in a medical setting. This type of stress test is called an *exercise stress test.*

During an exercise stress test, you are connected to an electrocardiograph machine and your electrocardiogram is continuously recorded. Your heart rate and blood pressure are also monitored very carefully, and a physician and nurse are always in attendance. Your performance throughout the test is carefully monitored. The chances of having a heart attack or dying during an exercise stress test are very low, on the order of 1 in 10,000 studies. Nevertheless, there are some risks associated with an exercise stress test. Patients who have had a recent heart attack or have frequent or unstable angina symptoms should not have an exercise stress test. Neither should patients with poorly controlled blood pressure or certain cardiac arrhythmias. Patients with certain heart valve disorders or an aortic aneurysm are at significantly increased risk during an exercise stress test. You must be evaluated by a physician to determine whether you are an appropriate candidate for an exercise stress test or any type of vigorous exercise regimen.

Many patients are fearful of this test, but a stress test is not a race, and running is not necessary. You don't need to be a star athlete, although some degree of coordination is necessary. If you can get on and off one of the moving walkways at the airport, you can probably walk

TABLE 5.1 *Exercise Levels for the Bruce Protocol*

Stage	Time (min)	Speed (mph)	Grade (%)	METS
I	3:00	1.7	10	5
II	6:00	2.5	12	7
III	9:00	3.4	14	9
IV	12:00	4.2	16	13
V	15:00	5.0	18	16

on a treadmill. During an exercise stress test, the treadmill's speed and degree of incline may vary. The Bruce protocol is the most common method employed, where the treadmill's speed and degree of incline are advanced every three minutes. The increasing levels of exercise make your body consume progressively greater degrees of oxygen, and in turn, progressively greater degrees of oxygen are demanded by your heart. The degree of oxygen consumption produced by the exercise is measured in metabolic equivalents (also called METs). One MET corresponds to the degree of oxygen consumption required to lie quietly in bed, two METs corresponds to twice that amount of oxygen consumption, and so on. Table 5.1 depicts the duration of exercise, treadmill speed, percentage grade of incline, and METs consumed for each level of a typical exercise stress test.

An exercise stress test is a rigorous test drive for your heart. It can produce a significant degree of oxygen consumption in a very short time. Your response to this test drive can tell your physician a great deal about the function of your heart, but like any test drive, it needs to last long enough to allow reliable observations. An inability to exercise for just a few minutes or an inability to increase your heart rate will limit the validity of the test. While an exercise stress test does not have a true finish line, there are predicted durations of exercise that are adjusted for age and gender. The duration of exercise is an important component of the test. This assessment of exercise capacity says a lot about the overall health of your body and will help your physician advise you as to what activities are appropriate for you. Table 5.2 provides several examples of common activities and the degree of METs required to complete them.

How your heart responds to the stress of exercise is an important

TABLE 5.2 *METs Required for Common Activities*

Activity	METs Required
Golfing with cart	2.5
Leisurely walking	3.3
Common household tasks	3.5
Mowing lawn	4.5
Chopping wood	3.9
Skiing (water or downhill)	6.8
Swimming	7.0
Jogging (10-minute mile)	10.2
Playing squash	12.1

Source: Fletcher et al., "Exercise Standards for Testing and Training," *Circulation* 104 (2001): 1720, table 8.

consideration. Both the heart rate and blood pressure are expected to increase with exercise. A heart rate that rises too rapidly with exercise suggests significant physical deconditioning. A heart rate that does not rise very much with exercise may reflect a medication you are taking or a problem with the electrical circuits in your heart. Drugs known as beta blockers commonly limit the heart rate response to exercise. A fall in blood pressure can be a worrisome development and could indicate a decline in your heart's pumping function during exercise. The physician supervising the test will decide whether to end or continue the stress test based on your physical signs during the test.

Thus far, we have discussed the physiological response to exercise. The clinical response to exercise is equally important. Clinical response generally means whether exercise is accompanied by any abnormal symptoms. Palpitations, any type of discomfort, or excessive shortness of breath can all indicate an underlying cardiac problem. The development of anginalike symptoms is suggestive but not diagnostic of coronary heart disease. As discussed previously, symptoms of angina can vary and are unreliable as an indication of myocardial ischemia. The diagnostic value of any exercise-induced symptoms (whether typical or atypical) increases significantly if there is other corroborative evidence of ongoing myocardial ischemia. Here the continuous recording of the electrocardiograph (EKG) is very helpful.

With a stress test, it is possible to monitor the heart's electrical

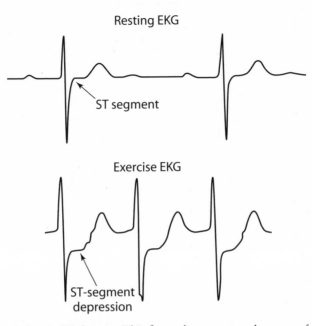

Resting EKG

ST segment

Exercise EKG

ST-segment
depression

FIGURE 5.2. Ischemic ST changes. This figure demonstrates the types of changes
in the EKG that are produced during a stress test given to a person with ischemia.
The upper panel depicts a normal EKG tracing. Note how the ST segment is
aligned with the baseline. The lower panel depicts significant depression of the
ST segment.

activity during exercise. Myocardial ischemia can induce alterations
in the way the heart is electrically activated. These changes are often
visualized as transient alterations in the electrocardiographic pattern.
The most common alteration is referred to as ST-segment depression.
Figure 5.2 depicts the transient type of ST-segment depression that
may occur during an exercise stress test.

The changes depicted in figure 5.2 are some of the more dramatic
ones. Others are far more subtle. These changes are even harder to
see if a person's baseline EKG is abnormal. A prior heart attack or
longstanding hypertension can result in permanent alterations of the
ST segment. In this setting, any exercise-induced ST changes are less
significant. Medications like digoxin or amiodarone can also induce
alterations of the ST segment without the person having any myocardial ischemia. Some people, women in particular, may develop

exercise-induced ST changes without any coronary heart disease at all. And in people who have a condition known as left bundle branch block, interpretation of ST-segment change is all but impossible. Thus, reliance solely on the observation of exercise-induced electrocardiographic changes may result in a number of falsely positive studies. A *false positive* here means exercise-induced alterations of the ST segment in the absence of significant coronary heart disease. Thus, sole reliance on the EKG is ill advised. The proper interpretation of an exercise stress test requires a thoughtful integration of the physiological response, the clinical response, and the electrocardiographic response to exercise. Taken collectively, these observations may allow your physician to determine more accurately whether you have obstructive coronary heart disease.

Picture a person who can exercise for an extended period. The heart rate and blood pressure rise normally and predictably. There are no symptoms with exercise, nor are there any electrocardiographic changes. Everyone would agree that the likelihood of this person having obstructive coronary heart disease is very low. Conversely, consider the patient who can exercise only a few minutes. At this low level of exercise, the heart rate becomes excessively high, and the blood pressure paradoxically falls. Chest discomfort and shortness of breath are associated with dramatic electrocardiographic changes. Here, too, everyone would agree: this patient has a high probability of having coronary heart disease. Wouldn't it be nice if all diagnoses were this easy?

They very often aren't easy, however, because between the two extreme cases just described, a multitude of ambiguous clinical situations exist. What happens, for example, if the patient is elderly or in poor shape and can't exercise very long? What happens if the patient is on medication preventing the heart rate and blood pressure from rising? What happens if the patient has had a prior heart attack and has an abnormal baseline electrocardiogram? Or if the patient has a condition that impairs the patient's ability to sense pain or produces chest pain by some mechanism other than myocardial ischemia? Or if there are exercise-related symptoms without any electrocardiographic changes?

As you can see, the standard exercise stress test can leave a lot of questions unanswered, and even when performed under the best of circumstances, standard exercise stress testing is of limited predictive value. It has a 65 to 70 percent sensitivity and specificity of detecting coronary heart disease. Said another way, a standard exercise stress test may miss up to 35 percent of the cases where significant atherosclerotic coronary obstruction is present. This may not seem too bad, unless this false negative is you or someone you know. Alternatively, a positive stress test does not necessarily indicate atherosclerotic heart disease. ST-segment changes may occur in various conditions that are unrelated to atherosclerosis. One of every three positive exercise tests will be a false positive. Given this high false positive and false negative rate, standard exercise stress testing is now considered wholly inadequate for the detection of coronary heart disease. There is a better way to look for atherosclerosis.

You may remember that in response to an increase in myocardial oxygen demand, coronary blood flow should increase three- to fivefold, because normal coronary arteries can dilate to increase their capacity for blood flow. An atherosclerotic coronary artery, on the other hand, has an impaired ability to augment its blood flow in response to the heart's call for more oxygen. Mildly diseased coronary arteries may be able to augment their flow to some degree, but a severely diseased coronary artery will not be able to augment its blood flow at all. It seems reasonable to ask whether the sensitivity and specificity of an exercise stress test could be increased if it could incorporate an assessment of the coronary blood flow response. This assessment is indeed possible, and it adds significant predictive value to an exercise stress test. Coronary blood flow assessment can be done noninvasively through nuclear imaging, a fairly simple concept.

Assessing Coronary Blood Flow

Picture a small river that branches into smaller streams. If you drop sand into the river and allow the current to carry the particles downstream, you will see that sand is deposited in locations in direct proportion to the amount of flow the areas receive. Areas with high flow get a lot of sand deposited. Areas with low flow get significantly less sand. The same thing occurs in the heart when you inject radioactive molecules into the bloodstream. Areas of the heart with lots of blood flow get lots of radioactive molecules deposited. Areas of the heart with less blood flow get fewer radioactive molecules. Just like particles of sand, the number of radioactive molecules that get deposited in your heart can be counted, and in doing so we can obtain a reasonably accurate assessment of which areas of the heart received more or less blood flow.

In reality, the number of radioactive molecules trapped within the heart is not actually counted. The radioactive molecules emit a very low level of radiation that can be quantified and converted into an image by a special type of camera. Because radioactive molecules are used, this test is sometimes referred to as a *nuclear imaging* or *nuclear stress test*. This isn't a very enticing or descriptive term. A more accurate term is a *myocardial perfusion scan*. The images obtained in a myocardial perfusion scan represent a map of the blood flow distribution (i.e., the perfusion) in the heart. If you are hunting for atherosclerosis, this is a useful map to have.

This myocardial perfusion scan is captured in a manner analogous to ultrafast CT scanning. Just before the stress test, a limited amount of radioactive tracer is administered intravenously. A camera then rotates around the body and acquires images of the heart from many different directions before the test and during it. The images are then reassembled and enhanced by computer to produce what is sometimes referred to as a single photon emission computed tomographic (SPECT) image. Both radioactive thallium and radioactive technetium have been used as the tracer molecules. In recent years, the technetium compounds have found increasing popularity because of their ability to produce sharper perfusion images. You may sometimes hear these imaging studies called Myoview or Cardiolite scans in reference to the brand name of the radioactive tracer used. The term *myocardial perfusion image*, however, is more descriptive and preferred.

Figure 5.3 shows several images from a myocardial perfusion scan. The myocardial perfusion images can be viewed on a monitor, stored in a computer, or printed on paper. Continuing with the sand analogy, consider that areas of the image that are viewed as being bright (i.e., emit lots of radioactivity) have high blood flow. Areas of

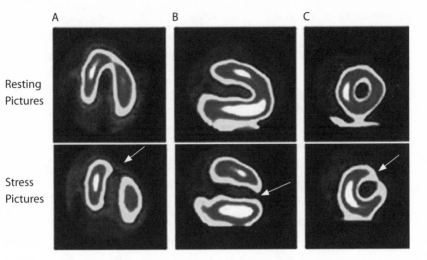

Resting Pictures

Stress Pictures

A   B   C

FIGURE 5.3.   Myocardial perfusion scan. This figure depicts nuclear myocardial perfusion images in a patient with obstructive coronary artery disease. The upper panels depict the myocardial perfusion pattern at rest. A homogenous perfusion pattern is seen in all myocardial segments. The lower panels depict the myocardial perfusion pattern during exercise. Note the prominent perfusion defects (absence of radioactivity, shown by arrows) seen during stress. This segment of the heart does not receive sufficient blood flow, which generally means that this segment is supplied by a critically narrowed coronary artery. Note that this type of scan does not provide information about which coronary artery is narrowed; nor does it provide information about how severely narrowed it is.

the heart that are less bright receive correspondingly less blood flow. The images provide an accurate map of the blood flow distribution in your heart.

In figure 5.3, notice that two sets of images are displayed. There is a reason for this. Recall that at rest, a person with coronary heart disease may have a normal blood flow distribution within the heart. This uniform blood flow distribution is depicted in the upper panels of figure 5.3. To visualize all areas of the heart, multiple views are obtained in various projections. Here, three cross-sectional images of the same heart are shown at rest. The heart is well outlined in each image, showing that all segments of this heart emit radioactivity. Compare these resting images with the three stress images. Notice how an abnormality in blood flow distribution only becomes apparent under stress conditions. This perfusion defect is depicted in the lower panels of figure 5.3 by the white arrows. This stress-induced perfusion defect involves a rather sizable segment of the heart. Based on the small amount of radioactivity present, there is little question that this segment of the heart does not receive sufficient blood flow under stress conditions. The patient almost certainly has coronary heart disease that limits the blood flow during exercise. The ability to detect abnormalities in blood flow distribution under stress conditions is more sensitive in detecting atherosclerotic disease than any component of a standard exercise stress test we have discussed.

Myocardial perfusion imaging, the ability to quantitate and visualize the blood flow within the heart, is one of the great advancements toward the diagnosis of coronary heart disease. The level of radiation emitted by the minute amounts of radioactive compounds injected into your body is quite low, roughly equivalent to that of a chest x-ray. You are not made "radioactive," and your radiation exposure is minimal. The radioactive life of the tracer is fairly short, and the tracer is eliminated from your body very quickly. Nonetheless, if you are pregnant, or could be pregnant, you should not have this test.

Myocardial perfusion imaging can actually do much more than assess the blood flow distribution within your heart. The test can provide additional important information about the viability of the heart muscle. Remember that the radioactive molecules need to be trapped by the heart muscle cells in order to be imaged by the nuclear camera. What happens if a portion of the heart muscle is damaged or scarred? Well the damaged heart muscle does not trap the radioactive molecules. They just flow on by. The absence of trapped radioactive molecules within the heart will appear as a "cold spot" on the resting perfusion scan *and* the stress perfusion scan. A persistent perfusion defect is indicative of a scarred heart muscle, or in other words, a prior heart attack. The perfusion scan can tell your physician with reasonable accuracy whether there has been damage to the heart, where it was, and how large the damage was. A myocardial perfusion scan can also identify viable but undersupplied areas of the heart that are likely to benefit from procedures designed to improve coronary blood flow.

Myocardial perfusion imaging has become an indispensable part of the stress test. With the addition of myocardial perfusion imaging, a stress test can detect coronary heart disease well over 90 percent of the time. A negative stress test with normal perfusion imaging is also of great value. It excludes the possibility of having significant atherosclerosis with a predictive accuracy of close to 98 percent. These tests, while not perfect, are extremely helpful in determining the presence or absence of coronary heart disease. Nonetheless, some caution in interpreting the tests is needed. In some instances, a perfusion image can be interpreted as normal when significant coronary heart disease is indeed present. Continued symptoms, despite a normal myocardial perfusion study, always require additional investigation.

Just as there are situations when the myocardial perfusion scan may be falsely negative, there are also situations when a myocardial perfusion scan may be falsely positive, suggesting that blood-flow-limiting coronary disease is present when it is not. A woman's breast, an elevated diaphragm, or abnormal lung tissue may all give the appearance of a perfusion defect on either resting or stress images. Thus, accurate interpretation of myocardial perfusion images must be coupled with the knowledge of functional capacity, clinical and physiological response to exercise, and whether there has been any alteration in the EKG. Taken together, an exercise stress test with myocardial perfusion imaging study are very powerful diagnostic tools for the detection of coronary heart disease.

In addition to understanding what type of information a myocardial perfusion image provides, it is important to understand what type of information it does *not* provide. A myocardial perfusion image enables the physician to *infer* that a portion of the heart may be supplied by a diseased, atherosclerotic artery. An inference, however, is nothing more than an educated guess. A myocardial perfusion scan does not tell the physician which vessel or vessels are narrowed. Nor does the perfusion scan indicate the degree of narrowing for a given vessel. The scan simply gives the physician an assessment of the relative blood flow distribution within the heart under the conditions of rest and exercise. From that assessment, the physician can develop a reasonable idea of whether a patient's heart is being supplied by normal or narrowed coronary arteries.

Because myocardial perfusion imaging adds considerable value to exercise stress testing, it should come as no surprise that James, given his recurrent indigestion and abnormal EKG, was scheduled to have an exercise test with perfusion imaging. But James was a young, healthy man. What happens to patients who cannot exercise because either they are too weak or they have a condition that prevents them from walking on a treadmill? Some patients may be limited by severe arthritis or poor circulation to the legs, for example. For patients who cannot exercise, a drug-induced, or pharmacological, stress test is a useful alternative. In fact, it's fairly easy to trick the heart into believing that the patient is exercising when the patient is sitting in a chair or lying on an examination table.

For a *pharmacological stress test,* a drug is administered to stimulate the heart temporarily into a state that is similar to an exercise-induced state. Though you aren't exercising, these drugs may make you feel a little flushed or jittery during the test. They may even produce angina or shortness of breath. These sensations last only a few minutes and are well tolerated by most people.

In a pharmacological stress test, the value of myocardial perfusion imaging is not decreased. It remains a very specific and sensitive test for the detection of coronary heart disease. The sensitivity and specificity of a positive pharmacological stress test is well over 90 percent, and a negative pharmacological stress test still confers an excellent prognosis. All that has changed with a pharmacological stress test is how the coronary blood flow is stimulated. It is done with an intravenous drug infusion rather than through exercise.

The most common way to perform a pharmacological stress test is to stimulate the heart with a brief intravenous infusion of a drug called adenosine. Adenosine is a short-acting but very powerful vasodilator that causes arteries to maximally dilate and thus increase their blood flow. When exposed to adenosine, the coronary arteries dilate as they do during intense exercise. Just as with an exercise stress test, a pharmacological stress test requires continuous monitoring with an EKG. A physician and a nurse are always in attendance. Perfusion images are obtained before and after the injection of the stress-producing drug. The images obtained of the resting and stress perfusion stages are every bit as good as the images obtained in an exercise stress test. One difference is that a pharmacological stress test does not allow us to assess the patient's functional capacity or physiological response to exercise. Because this type of test is generally performed only when the patient is already *known* to have impaired exercise capacity, however, this difference is of little or no significance.

A pharmacological stress test with adenosine is fairly safe for many patients, but it certainly is not a test recommended for everyone. Some other medications may block the actions of adenosine, preventing the vasodilation that is required to duplicate the conditions of stress. Aminophylline, a medication commonly used to treat asthma, completely blocks the actions of adenosine. If you are taking aminophylline or aminophylline-like medications, you cannot have an adenosine-mediated stress test. Other medications, like dipyridamole (Persantine), may dangerously prolong the actions of adenosine. Dipyridamole is sometimes used to treat mild stroke or poor circulation in the legs. If you are taking any form of dipyridamole, you cannot have an adenosine stress test. Other situations where an adenosine stress test is contraindicated (inadvisable) include very low blood pressure and blocked heart valves. Intravenous adenosine administration causes the blood pressure temporarily to fall and the heart rate to slow in almost everyone, so patients with too low a blood pressure or too slow a heart rate to begin with cannot tolerate adenosine. In certain conditions, the heart valves are blocked or the blood vessels supplying the brain are narrowed to a degree that makes the use of intravenous adenosine unsafe.

For people who are able to tolerate a brief adenosine infusion, the pharmacological stress test is a viable alternative to exercise stress testing. For people who can't, an intravenous infusion of the drug dobutamine is sometimes used. Dobutamine is high-octane fuel for the heart. It causes your heart to beat faster and harder, just like during exercise. With a dobutamine stress test, as with other stress tests, perfusion images are obtained before and after an intravenous infusion of the drug. Either intravenous adenosine or intravenous dobutamine can be used to perform a pharmacological stress test with myocardial perfusion imaging. The doctor performing the stress test will be the best judge of which drug is best for a particular patient.

A stress test (whether it is exercise induced or pharmacologically induced) with myocardial perfusion imaging is the most common method of looking for coronary heart disease, but there are several other ways to detect myocardial ischemia during a stress test. You may remember that when a portion of the heart receives insufficient blood flow during exercise, it may not contract normally. This stress-induced *wall motion abnormality* may be visualized several ways. The most common way is to image the heart with ultrasound.

Seeing the Heart with Sound

The technology employed by echocardiography is similar to that used by sonar for submarine navigation. High-frequency sound waves can penetrate the chest wall and bounce off the heart. The resulting echo can then be reconstructed by computer to form an image of the heart. The image is captured in real time and can show motion of the heart's walls and valves with each beat. The echocardiogram can provide an excellent representation of the heart's size and contracting ability. And an echocardiogram can be coupled with a stress test to hunt for atherosclerotic disease.

Rather than examining blood flow distribution before and after stress, a stress echocardiogram examines the heart's contracting ability. As with myocardial perfusion images, echocardiographic images of the heart are obtained at rest and during periods of stress. A comparison is then made between the two images with respect to the heart's wall motion under both conditions. A normal heart uniformly increases its contracting ability with exercise. A heart supplied by atherosclerotic coronary arteries may show regions that minimally contract or perhaps do not contract at all. Once again, in the regions where the wall motion is abnormal, the inference is that atherosclerotic coronary arteries are limiting the amount of blood flow during periods of stress. Much like a myocardial perfusion scan, the stress echocardiogram can be performed with exercise-induced stress or by infusing a drug such as dobutamine.

The development of stress-induced wall motion abnormalities is very specific for coronary heart disease. A stress echocardiogram can be every bit as sensitive and specific as a myocardial perfusion scan. Its positive predictive value is well over 90 percent, and a negative study carries an excellent prognosis. Properly done and interpreted, it can be an excellent test in the right patients. Unfortunately, stress echocardiographic images can have considerable variability. Some people, because of their shape or size, are not good candidates for the test. It may be difficult for the ultrasound waves to penetrate their chest wall and produce images that can be reliably interpreted. As with all tests described in this chapter, a stress echocardiogram is not for everyone.

Regardless of your age, shape, or size, there is a stress test that is right for you. Your doctor will know which one is best. What is important to remember is that exercise stress tests with either myocardial perfusion imaging or wall motion analysis by echocardiography are powerful tools for diagnosing coronary heart disease.

Our patient James had an exercise stress test with myocardial perfusion imaging. Shortly after James began exercising, his indigestion returned. The EKG recorded striking ST-segment depression with exercise that eventually resolved with rest. The myocardial perfusion images revealed a large perfusion defect on the anterior surface of the heart; it, too, resolved with rest. By every criteria, James had an abnormal stress test, and he had a very high likelihood of having significant obstruction of one or more of his coronary arteries. In fact, some features of his stress test suggested that he was in an unfavorable prognostic category. Additional testing was now in order. Knowing the full extent to which atherosclerotic disease has invaded James's heart will help his physician decide which therapeutic options are best for him.

The most common means of refining the information from an abnormal stress test is to visualize all the coronary arteries during their course through the heart. This can be very difficult to do because the coronary arteries are very small and their path through the heart is tortuous. And they are moving back and forth sixty to ninety times per minute! Ultrafast CT scanning provides a glimpse of the coronary arteries, but its resolution is not clear enough to accurately assess the degree of arterial narrowing. The only way to visualize these tiny blood vessels accurately is to fill them with a radio-opaque substance and then take high-speed motion pictures with x-rays. A movie clip of the heart's blood vessels obtained this way is commonly referred to as a *coronary arteriogram*.

What Does Coronary Arteriography Add?

Although plain x-rays easily penetrate soft tissues, the demarcation between adjacent structures is often indistinct. As a result, it is impossible for plain x-rays to reveal the extent of coronary heart disease. To visualize an outline of the coronary arteries accurately with x-rays, the arteries need to be temporarily filled with a radio-opaque material sometimes referred to as "dye." The material isn't dye, however; it is a clear liquid containing iodine molecules. This material is injected directly into the coronary arteries. The x-rays are blocked by the iodine molecules in the contrast material, allowing the blood vessels to appear as opaque lines in the movie clip. Since only the coronary arteries contain the contrast agent, they are the only structures that block the x-rays, producing crisp and very clear images of the entire coronary arterial tree. Figure 5.4 depicts angiographic images of both normal (a) and highly atherosclerotic (b) coronary arteries.

Coronary arteriography is extremely useful. In figure 5.4a, notice how smooth the normal coronary arteries are. You can easily see how theses "pipes" are able to carry the blood supply to the heart muscle in an unimpeded manner. In figure 5.4b, notice how the coronary arteries are severely narrowed in multiple locations. Remember that the diameter of these vessels is only a few millimeters. The arrows in figure 5.4b identify two narrowings that have reduced the diameter of the left anterior descending coronary artery by over 95 percent. For a three-millimeter blood vessel, this means that the remaining channel through the coronary artery is only a few tenths of a millimeter in diameter. The heart muscle supplied by this highly diseased artery is literally hanging by a thread. The type of narrowing depicted in figure 5.4b requires an urgent intervention.

As you can see, in a coronary arteriogram, only the coronary arteries are visualized. It is important that no other structures obstruct their view. The only way to ensure that the coronary arteries and only the coronary arteries are completely opacified is to inject the contrast material directly into the coronary artery. This is done by advancing a small flexible tube called a *catheter* up to the heart and ultimately into the coronary arteries. The iodine contrast agent is then administered

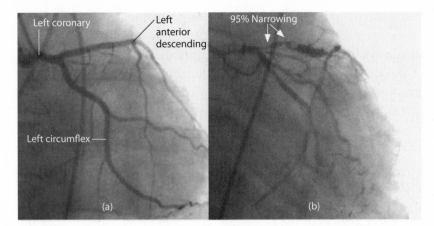

FIGURE 5.4. Angiographic images of (a) normal coronary arteries and (b) athero-sclerotic coronary arteries. A 95 percent narrowing of the left anterior descend-ing coronary artery is identified by the white arrows in (b). In addition, a promi-nent filling defect appears within the left anterior descending coronary artery. This finding represents partially obstructive coronary thrombus. Multiple other segments of coronary artery disease are present in (b) but are not highlighted.

via a small injection. Because visualizing the coronary arteries in-volves the use of this small catheter, the procedure is sometimes called *cardiac catheterization*. The procedure we have discussed, however, involves taking pictures of the coronary arteries. Accordingly, coro-nary arteriography is a more accurate and preferred term. In reality, coronary arteriography may be only one part of a cardiac catheteriza-tion. During a cardiac catheterization procedure, the small tube can be advanced to many different locations in the heart for the injection of contrast and for the selective imaging of other chambers or blood vessels. The catheter may also be used to obtain measurements of blood pressure and flow at various locations in the heart. In this book, we will be discussing only the part of the cardiac catheterization pro-cedure pertaining to coronary arteriography.

For many people, the thought of inserting a small tube into the heart is understandably frightening. (The potential complications of this test are discussed later in this chapter.) If you are going to have this procedure, it may help you to know exactly how it works. A cardiac catheterization is always performed at a hospital by a physician specially trained to do this type of procedure. In a room similar to an operating room, you are attended to by a team of nurses who attach electrocardiograph leads that continuously monitor your heart. A device called a *pulse oximeter,* similar to a clothespin, is placed on your finger to monitor the oxygen content of your blood, and an intravenous line is inserted into your vein to facilitate the administration of medications. A cardiac catheterization laboratory is a very safe environment, and the test itself, while it carries some risk (see below), is reasonably safe. Nonetheless, many patients are anxious about the procedure, and most patients are given a mild sedative.

To access the coronary arteries, the catheter must enter one of the larger arteries in the body and then be manually advanced to the heart. The most common site of entry is the femoral artery in the groin, although access can also be obtained through the radial artery in the wrist or the brachial artery near the elbow. The area where the catheter is to be inserted is first prepared by a sterile scrub. The skin and surrounding tissues are then infiltrated with a local anesthetic. Once the area is anesthetized, the artery is entered with a small needle. The catheter is then advanced through the insertion site. A surgical incision is not required.

The catheter that is used is small, only one to two millimeters in diameter. Since there are no nerve endings inside the blood vessels, the passage of the catheter from the insertion site to the heart is completely painless. The physician performing the procedure uses x-ray images that are displayed on the monitor to help guide the movement of the catheter. Many patients marvel as they watch the catheter's advance on the monitor. Depending what additional procedures are being performed, a coronary arteriogram may take anywhere from fifteen minutes to over an hour. At the conclusion of the procedure, the catheter is simply withdrawn through the hole by which it was inserted. Some pressure is then applied to the access site to prevent bleeding. A small bandage is applied, and the procedure is complete. Most patients are observed in the hospital for several hours after the procedure to ensure that there is no additional bleeding from the insertion site. The overwhelming majority of patients are discharged home the same day.

Despite continuing improvements in noninvasive cardiac imaging, coronary arteriography is considered the gold standard for directly visualizing the coronary arteries. A coronary arteriogram will clearly identify which coronary arteries have atherosclerotic narrowing. In general, the degree of coronary arterial narrowing is visually estimated by the physician and reported as a percent reduction in the vessel diameter. A 70 percent stenosis means that the internal diameter of the coronary artery is reduced by 70 percent. It is important to remember that the *reduction* in diameter is compared to the diameter of a "normal" segment of vessel. This comparative technique is limited by the ability to find a segment of artery that is truly normal and can thus serve as an accurate basis for comparison.

In patients with diffuse atherosclerotic disease, this comparative nature of reporting may actually underestimate the severity of their atherosclerosis. This may be particularly true in people with diabetes, who tend to develop a diffuse narrowing throughout the coronary arterial tree. Another limitation of coronary arteriography is that while it provides an *anatomical* description of the atherosclerotic disease, it does not provide any information about whether the observed coronary stenosis is actually limiting blood flow and thus whether it may be responsible for the patient's symptoms. This is why it is important to correlate the findings of the coronary arteriogram with a *physiological* study, such as a stress test.

In general (but not always), a stenosis that exhibits a greater than 70 percent diameter reduction is believed to be physiologically significant (flow-limiting). Excellent laboratory data and clinical data support this physiological benchmark. When assessing the severity of coronary stenosis, a 70 percent diameter reduction has become the threshold for guiding most clinical decisions regarding the need for intervention.

Not all coronary stenoses that exceed a 70 percent diameter reduction are responsible for symptoms of angina. The heart has a wonderful way of accommodating to a slowly progressing coronary stenosis. It can develop alternative channels, called *collateral arteries,* to allow blood to flow around a narrowed coronary artery. The collateral arteries are generally quite small but can provide an alternative blood supply to a jeopardized area of the heart. Under most conditions, this alternative blood supply is sufficient to minimize or even

TABLE 5.3 *Complications of Coronary Arteriography*

Death, myocardial infarction, or neurological event	0.12%
Nonfatal arrhythmias	0.3%
Local vascular problem requiring surgical repair	1.6%
Nonfatal allergic reaction	2.0%
Transient decline in renal function	5.0%
Renal failure requiring dialysis	<1.0%

Source: Adapted from *Cardiac Catheterization, Arteriography, and Intervention,* ed. Donald S. Baim and William Grossman (Baltimore, Md.: Williams & Wilkins, 1996), 18.

prevent the symptoms of angina. At high levels of exercise, however, when the need for an increased blood supply is greatest, the blood supplied by the collaterals may be insufficient, and thus the person develops anginal symptoms. Collateral blood vessels are good because they can reduce the physiological significance of obstructive coronary artery disease, but they are not the perfect alternative to natural coronary arteries. You can think of the collateral vessels as being a detour around a blocked interstate highway. While the alternative path may eventually enable you to reach your destination, it is nowhere near as good as the major highway you started out on.

Coronary arteriography is unquestionably a valuable tool in the diagnosis and management of patients with coronary heart disease, but a coronary arteriogram is not needed for nor should it be performed in every person with suspected atherosclerosis. While generally safe, it is an invasive test and carries the risk of significant complications, including the possibility of death (see table 5.3).

When performed by an experienced physician, a coronary arteriogram is a reasonably safe procedure. The overall risk of dying is less than 1 in 1,000 (0.1 percent risk). Because the catheter enters the aorta and the blood vessels in the heart, there is a low risk of stroke, heart attack, or alteration in cardiac rhythm. The actual risk to any patient may be somewhat higher or lower, depending on the patient's age and medical conditions.

One of the most common complications of coronary arteriography is related to persistent bleeding at the arterial puncture site, which occurs in about 5 percent of patients. In older people, in obese people, or in those who have been taking anticoagulants, the risk of bleeding may be somewhat higher. In most cases, the bleeding is manifest as a large bruise (called a *hematoma*) at the insertion site. The hematoma generally resolves on its own in about a week to ten days. In some people, the leak persists or an enlargement in the artery called a *pseudoaneruysm* forms. Between 1 and 2 percent of patients require a blood transfusion or surgical repair of the pseudoaneruysm. Because of this small risk, it is essential that all patients who have had a coronary arteriogram be seen by their physician one to two weeks after the procedure. Infections at the insertion site are rare. Patients with heart murmurs or artificial heart valves generally do not require antibiotic prophylaxis prior to this procedure.

The coronary arteriogram procedure also carries some risk that pertains to the contrast agent used. Some patients are allergic to compounds containing iodine and react adversely to the iodine contrast agent. Approximately 2 percent of patients have this reaction, which is rarely life threatening. There is currently no alternative to using the iodine-based contrast agent. Patients who are allergic to iodine can still undergo coronary arteriography. If you believe that you may be allergic to iodine, you should mention this concern to your physician prior to the procedure, and he or she may be able to medicate you to prevent any allergic reaction.

The iodine-based contrast agent is eliminated from the body by the kidneys. The ability to excrete this agent is impaired if you have any form of kidney disease. In fact, in patients with preexisting kidney disease, the contrast agent may temporarily worsen kidney function. Rarely, this problem can progress to the point where the patient requires dialysis. If you have any form of kidney disease, discuss the possibility of worsening kidney function with your doctor before the procedure. Some medications, especially metformin (which is a drug frequently used to treat diabetes), may increase the risk of kidney dysfunction following coronary arteriography. This medication is commonly discontinued for a short period before and after the procedure. Administering intravenous fluids before, during, and after the test helps assure a continuous and brisk urine output and is of great value in minimizing, though not eliminating, the risk of kidney problems. The administration of medications such as N-acetylcysteine

(Mucomyst) prior to administering iodine contrast agents has also been shown to be of some benefit.

Because coronary arteriography does entail some risks, it should be performed only when there are clear indications to do so. As noted previously, it is possible to use a catheter to examine many parts of the heart. For the purposes of detecting the presence of atherosclerosis, however, only visualization of the coronary arteries is needed. The common indications for coronary arteriography are listed in table 5.4.

James's indications for coronary arteriography were clear. The EKG suggested that he had sustained a prior heart attack. He developed indigestion with minimal activity. His stress test was very abnormal and suggestive of an unfavorable prognostic category. It was clear that additional information regarding his coronary anatomy was required not only to outline his risk for future cardiac events but also to determine which of the various therapeutic options was best for him. James was scheduled for a coronary arteriogram that week. Given the very high probability that he had significant coronary heart disease, his doctor prescribed several different medications for James to begin taking in the meantime.

TABLE 5.4   *Common Indications for Coronary Arteriography*

all patients with noninvasive-testing evidence suggestive of a high risk for future cardiovascular events

patients who are on medications and remain symptomatic with minimal activity

survivors of a cardiac arrest or patients with evidence of life-threatening cardiac arrhythmias

patients with an unstable pattern of angina pectoris or those who exhibit evidence of myocardial damage consistent with an acute coronary syndrome

patients with congestive heart failure and symptoms of angina or patients with ventricular dysfunction for whom noninvasive studies suggest the presence of underlying atherosclerotic heart disease

patients during the acute phase of a myocardial infarction

patients who experience angina symptoms early after a myocardial infarction

patients who experience angina within nine months after a coronary intervention procedure

Source: Condensed and adapted from *Braunwald's Heart Disease: A Textbook of Cardiovascular Medicine,* ed. Eugene Braunwald et al., 7th ed. (Philadelphia: Elsevier Saunders, 2005), 396.

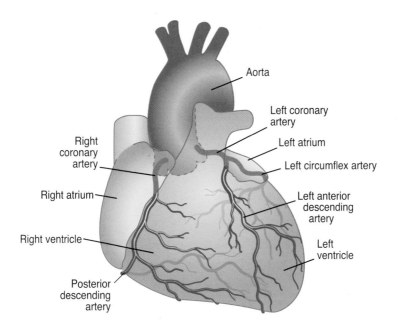

Aorta

Left coronary artery

Right coronary artery

Left atrium

Left circumflex artery

Right atrium

Left anterior descending artery

Right ventricle

Left ventricle

Posterior descending artery

PLATE 1. Heart with coronary arteries (from the front). The human heart is roughly the size of a man's fist. It has four separate chambers pumping blood: the right atrium (RA) and right ventricle (RV), and the left atrium (LA) and left ventricle (LV), which pump blood to the brain and rest of the body. The heart receives its blood supply via branches of the aorta called coronary arteries. The right coronary artery (RCA) supplies the right ventricle and lower surface of the left ventricle. The left anterior descending (LAD) coronary artery and left circumflex (LCX) coronary artery supply most of the left ventricle. Blood exiting the left ventricle travels through the aorta. In the aortic arch, large blood vessels supplying the brain, the carotid arteries, emerge.

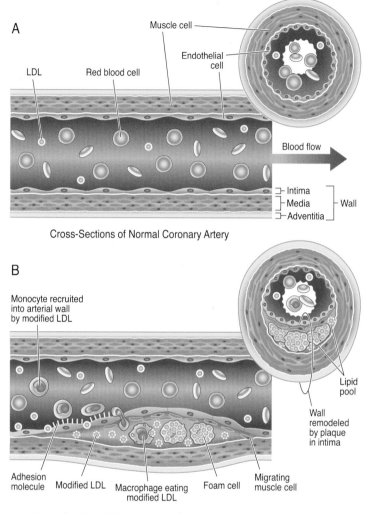

A

Muscle cell

Endothelial cell

LDL Red blood cell

Blood flow

Intima
Media } Wall
Adventitia

Cross-Sections of Normal Coronary Artery

B

Monocyte recruited
into arterial wall
by modified LDL

Lipid
pool

Wall
remodeled
by plaque
in intima

Adhesion
molecule Modified LDL Macrophage eating
modified LDL Foam cell Migrating
muscle cell

Cross-Sections of Atherosclerotic Coronary Artery

PLATE 2. (A) Longitudinal and cross-section view of a normal coronary artery. This part of the figure depicts a smooth blood vessel channel and the unobstructed flow of blood. Notice the thin blood vessel wall composed of three layers: the intima, media, and adventitia. (B) Longitudinal and cross-section view of an atherosclerotic artery. Note how components of the blood have migrated into the blood vessel wall to form a lipid pool between the intima and adventitia layers. This part of the figure demonstrates how the atherosclerotic *process* not only narrows the blood vessel channel but also damages and remodels the arterial wall.

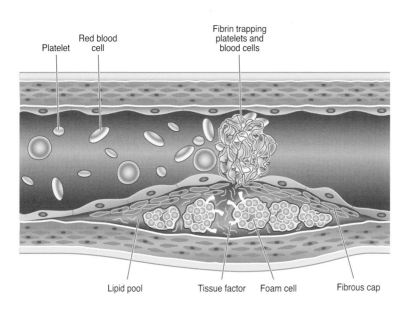

Platelet   Red blood cell   Fibrin trapping platelets and blood cells

Lipid pool   Tissue factor   Foam cell   Fibrous cap

PLATE 3. Atherosclerotic plaque rupture. Shown is the essential feature in the transformation of a stable atherosclerotic plaque into an unstable one. Here, rupture of the fibrous cap allows a blood clot, composed of fibrin and platelets, to form. Left untreated, this thrombus may grow to occlude the artery, disrupting blood flow.

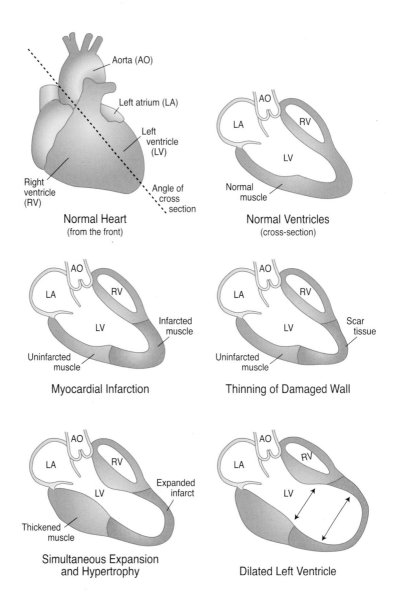

Normal Heart
(from the front)

Aorta (AO)

Left atrium (LA)

Left ventricle (LV)

Right ventricle (RV)

Angle of cross section

Normal Ventricles
(cross-section)

AO
LA
RV
LV
Normal muscle

Myocardial Infarction

AO
LA
RV
LV
Infarcted muscle
Uninfarcted muscle

Thinning of Damaged Wall

AO
LA
RV
LV
Scar tissue
Uninfarcted muscle

Simultaneous Expansion and Hypertrophy

AO
LA
RV
LV
Expanded infarct
Thickened muscle

Dilated Left Ventricle

AO
LA
RV
LV

PLATE 4. Cardiac remodeling. After a myocardial infarction (a heart attack), the infarcted muscle begins to thin. In response to the intracardiac blood pressure, the thin and weakened tissue begins to expand. Simultaneously, the uninfarcted cardiac segments begin to contract more vigorously, resulting in thickening, or hypertrophy. Over time, the combination of infarct expansion and wall hypertrophy causes the left ventricular cavity to dilate. This change is manifest as an enlarged and weakened heart that functions less efficiently. The cardiac remodeling sets the stage for the development of congestive heart failure, cardiac arrhythmia, and stroke.

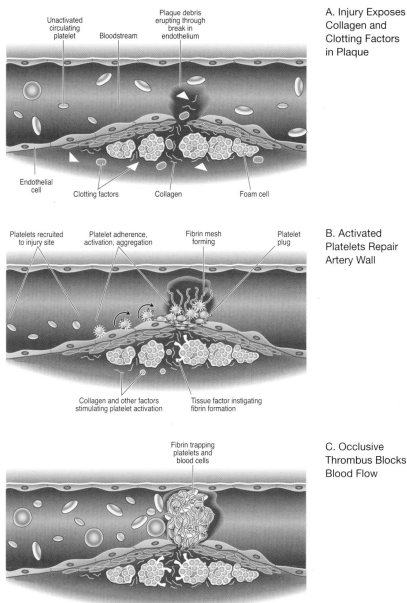

A. Injury Exposes Collagen and Clotting Factors in Plaque

Unactivated circulating platelet

Bloodstream

Plaque debris erupting through break in endothelium

Endothelial cell

Clotting factors

Collagen

Foam cell

B. Activated Platelets Repair Artery Wall

Platelets recruited to injury site

Platelet adherence, activation, aggregation

Fibrin mesh forming

Platelet plug

Collagen and other factors stimulating platelet activation

Tissue factor instigating fibrin formation

C. Occlusive Thrombus Blocks Blood Flow

Fibrin trapping platelets and blood cells

PLATE 5. Transformation of a stable atherosclerotic plaque into an unstable one. (A) Injury to the endothelial lining exposes the contents of the blood vessel wall to circulating blood products. This interaction sets the stage for activation of the blood coagulation system and platelet activation and aggregation. (B) Platelets, circulating in the blood, adhere to the site of injury, where they interact with collagen and clotting factors to become activated. Activated platelets also adhere to the site of injury, aggregating additional platelets and fibrin to form a fibrin mesh and platelet plug. (C) The platelet plug and fibrin mesh trap additional platelets and blood products to form an occlusive thrombus (blood clot).

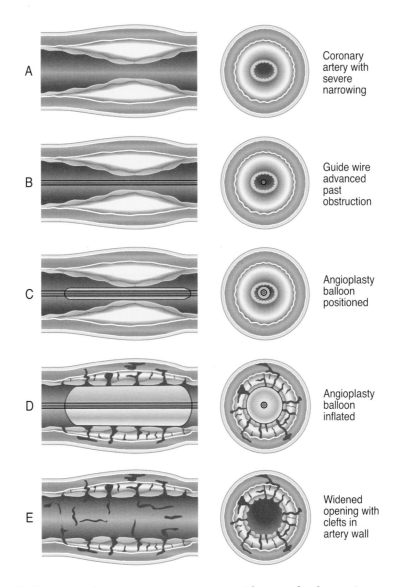

A — Coronary artery with severe narrowing

B — Guide wire advanced past obstruction

C — Angioplasty balloon positioned

D — Angioplasty balloon inflated

E — Widened opening with clefts in artery wall

PLATE 6. Balloon angioplasty. (A) A coronary artery with severe focal stenosis (note the very small open channel in the blood vessel). (B) A guide wire measuring 0.014 inches in diameter is threaded through the stenosis. (C) The angioplasty balloon is advanced over the guide wire and positioned so that it straddles the stenotic region. (D) The angioplasty balloon is inflated, producing many small clefts in the blood vessel wall. (E) The angioplasty balloon and guide wire are withdrawn, revealing significant improvement in the lumen diameter. Many deep clefts remain in the blood vessel wall, however, and they are potent stimuli for thrombus formation.

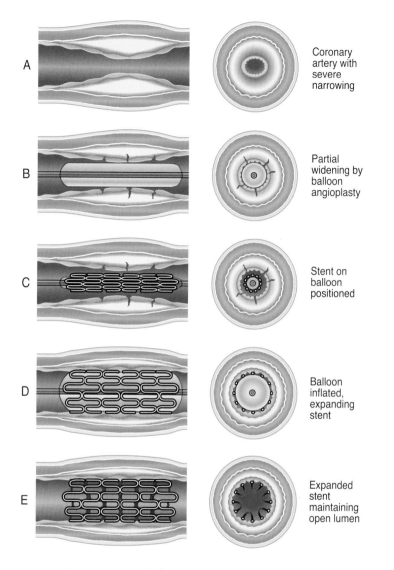

A — Coronary artery with severe narrowing

B — Partial widening by balloon angioplasty

C — Stent on balloon positioned

D — Balloon inflated, expanding stent

E — Expanded stent maintaining open lumen

PLATE 7. Coronary stent deployment. (A) A coronary artery with severe focal stenosis. (B) The stenosis is partially predilated with balloon angioplasty. A 0.014-inch guide wire remains in place. (C) An unexpanded coronary stent is placed on an angioplasty balloon and positioned so that it straddles the stenotic region. (D) The balloon is inflated, expanding the stent and embedding it in the blood vessel wall. (E) The balloon and guide wire are removed, leaving the fully deployed coronary stent in place. Note how the vessel lumen has been enlarged and the clefts on the arterial wall obliterated. The exposed metal struts of the stent remain in contact with the blood and may be the stimuli for future thrombus formation.

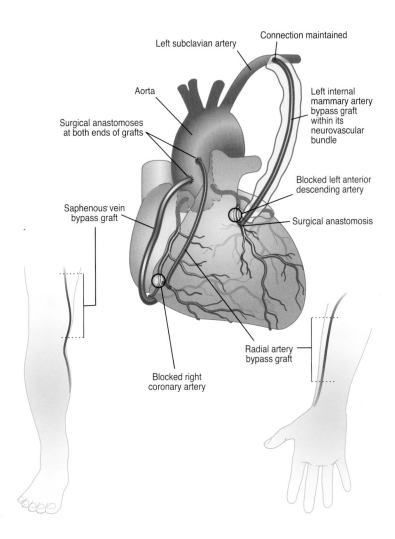

Left subclavian artery

Connection maintained

Aorta

Left internal mammary artery bypass graft within its neurovascular bundle

Surgical anastomoses at both ends of grafts

Blocked left anterior descending artery

Saphenous vein bypass graft

Surgical anastomosis

Radial artery bypass graft

Blocked right coronary artery

PLATE 8. Coronary artery bypass grafts. The types of conduits used in a triple-vessel coronary bypass surgery are shown. An internal mammary artery graft extends from the left subclavian artery to the coronary artery, past the site of coronary artery obstruction. Note how the internal mammary artery graft maintains its original upstream connection with the arterial system. The downstream connection is made with microscopic sutures, forming a *surgical anastomosis*. Also note how the neurovascular bundle associated with this artery is preserved throughout the course of the bypass graft. Radial artery and saphenous vein bypass grafts are distinctly different in that they require separate connections (anastomoses) to both the aorta and the coronary artery, which means that their neurovascular bundles are not kept intact.

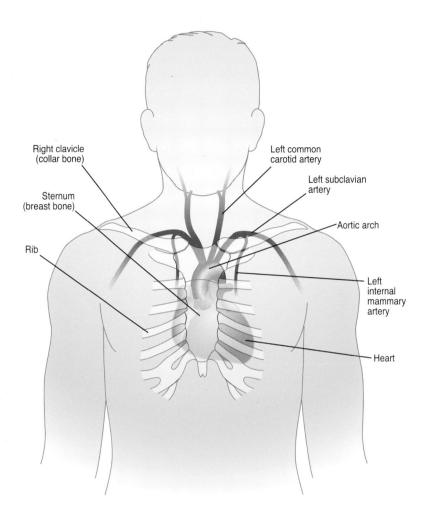

Right clavicle
(collar bone)

Left common
carotid artery

Left subclavian
artery

Sternum
(breast bone)

Aortic arch

Rib

Left
internal
mammary
artery

Heart

PLATE 9. Major branches of the aortic arch. Blood exits the heart via the aorta, traveling throughout the body. Arising from the aortic arch are large blood vessels supplying the brain and upper extremities. The carotid arteries are the major blood supply to the brain. The subclavian arteries are the major blood supply to the arms. The sternum and ribs lie just above the aortic arch, and these bony structures are supplied by branches of the internal mammary arteries.

SIX

What Are All These Medications For?

....

James left the doctor's office with a fist full of prescriptions, a bag full of medication samples, and a mind full of questions. Two weeks ago he'd thought he was a healthy man. Now he was taking a smorgasbord of medications with a list of side effects as long as his arm. James wanted to know more about these medications: Why so many? What do they do? And what about side effects? This chapter is designed to answer these questions.

Why does one condition require so many different medications? The answer, as we have seen, is that coronary heart disease has many different components. Controlling this disease requires taking measures to prevent the formation of blood clots, to reduce inflammation of the blood vessels, and to inhibit cholesterol formation and transport within the body. And these efforts are designed only to prevent further advancement of atherosclerosis. Once atherosclerosis has progressed to the point where it produces symptoms, therapies are needed to enable the heart to work more efficiently and accommodate to the reduction in coronary blood flow. This chapter explores the complex *medical management* (i.e., through medication, not surgery or other invasive procedures) of atherosclerosis (coronary heart disease).

Preventing the formation of a coronary thrombus—a blood clot—is one of the foundations of medical therapy for atherosclerosis. When we scrape our skin, the bleeding eventually stops because the body's coagulation system is activated and a clot forms over the injured area. As we saw in chapters 2 and 3, while clotting may be good for an injury to the skin, it is not good for an injury to the lining of a blood vessel. Blood clots are instrumental in the development of symptomatic coronary heart disease. Adhering to atherosclerotic plaque, a blood clot may abruptly obstruct the entire blood vessel, causing a heart attack, or slowly narrow the inner channel of an artery, causing symptoms of angina. Thus, medications to prevent clot formation help prevent angina symptoms by altering the process that leads to the obstruction of the coronary artery. In doing so, these medications may prevent not only the symptoms of angina but also the progression of these symptoms into a full-blown heart attack.

Preventing Clots with Platelet Inhibitors

A thrombus is composed of two main components: platelets and fibrin. These components of thrombus usually circulate in the bloodstream in an inactive state, but if they are activated by any number of different circulating clotting factors, platelets and fibrin may form a blood clot. Because platelets, fibrin, and the various clotting factors all interact to form a thrombus, we must interrupt their interaction to help prevent the formation of clots. Anticoagulants are an important part of treating coronary heart disease because they work to interrupt the interaction of these elements.

Platelets are blood cells, and like all blood cells, they are formed in the bone marrow. They begin their life as part of much larger cells called *megakaryocytes*. As megakaryocytes enter the bloodstream, they break into the little chemical packets called platelets. Platelets travel throughout the body in an inactive state. They circulate in the bloodstream like pieces of confetti, ready to stick to an injured site and initiate blood clot formation. In blood vessels, damage to the endothelial lining allows the platelets to be exposed to collagen and other clotting factors in the inner layers of the blood vessel wall. This exposure to "foreign" material causes the platelets to adhere to the site of injury, just like when you scrape your knee—except in this instance, the process is happening inside the coronary artery.

Once the platelets adhere, they soon become activated, changing their shape and disgorging their chemical contents in the vicinity of the vascular injury. The local release of these platelet factors stimulates more platelet aggregation and more platelet activation, causing a chain reaction that leads to the formation of a *platelet plug*. Mountains of platelets soon form at the site of endothelial damage, producing a seal that promotes the healing process (see plate 5).

Platelet aggregation and platelet activation are rapid and self-propagating processes. Platelet aggregation stimulates platelet activation; platelet activation stimulates platelet aggregation; and so on. The first step in treating active coronary heart disease is preventing thrombus formation by inhibiting the many chemical factors involved in this aggregation and activation process.

Inflammation of the coronary artery wall is another important element of active atherosclerosis. This inflammation is an intravascular inflammatory response that helps fuel the atherosclerotic process by damaging the endothelial lining, which in turn initiates thrombus formation, and so on. Inflammation also stimulates platelet activation. The link between inflammation and platelet activation is a compound called *thromboxane A2*. Thromboxane A2 is generated during the inflammatory process that characterizes atherosclerosis. Thus, inhibiting the formation of thromboxane A2 is a significant part of medical management.

A reduction in thromboxane A2 decreases the degree of inflammation in the atherosclerotic plaque, making it less likely that a plaque will rupture and cause a heart attack. Any reduction in thromboxane A2 formation will limit the degree of platelet activation at the site of an atherosclerotic plaque, and reducing platelet activation at the site of an atherosclerotic plaque will in turn decrease the chance of forming an occlusive thrombus. The result will be fewer unstable angina symptoms and a lower incidence of heart attack. There is one medication that will decrease both inflammation and platelet aggregation. It's plain old aspirin.

Thromboxane A2 formation can be impaired by taking aspirin or drugs known as nonsteroidal anti-inflammatory drugs (NSAIDs). Thromboxane A2 is formed through a chemical reaction involving a family of enzymes called *cyclooxygenase* (COX). There are two cyclooxygenase enzymes, COX 1 and COX 2, and aspirin inhibits the action of both. By inhibiting the COX enzymes, aspirin reduces the amount of thromboxane A2 that is formed. Less thromboxane A2 means less inflammation and less platelet activation.

Unfortunately, aspirin has other actions as well. Inhibiting COX 1 also reduces the amount of protective secretions lining the stomach, increasing the risk of gastric irritation and ulcer formation. Without normally functioning platelets, there is an increased risk of gastrointestinal bleeding. The potential benefits of aspirin therapy, then, must be weighed in the context of the relative risk for coronary heart disease and the relative risk for bleeding or another aspirin-related complication. Your doctor can help weigh the risks and benefits for you. Although aspirin is available over the counter, it has some very potent effects. You should not take aspirin regularly without the advice and consent of your doctor.

Gastric irritation and risk of significant bleeding makes nonspecific COX inhibitors a bad choice for some people. In recent years, a group of agents were developed that inhibit only the COX 2 enzyme. These *selective COX 2 inhibitors* held great promise. In theory, these drugs would inhibit only COX 2, the portion of the COX pathway that was responsible for inflammation, without affecting the secretion of protective gastric mucous (COX 1). The COX 2 inhibitors—rofecoxib (Vioxx), celecoxib (Celebrex), and valdecoxib (Bextra)—certainly lived up to expectations as potent anti-inflammatory medications with few gastric side effects. They were very effective in treating arthritis, an inflammatory disease.

Several clinical trials designed to assess the efficacy of these drugs in treating people with arthritis noted an increased incidence of heart attack, and there is considerable controversy over the safety of these medications for people with coronary heart disease. Rofecoxib and valdecoxib have been withdrawn from the market, and cautions have been issued about the use of celecoxib in people with coronary heart disease. What causes the increased incidence of heart attack in people taking theses drugs is not entirely clear. We have all been in the situation where one highway becomes blocked and all alternate roads become congested with additional traffic. It is possible that, similarly, by inhibiting just one of the COX enzymes (COX 2), the other arm of the chemical pathway (COX 1) becomes overloaded, permitting the accumulation of substances that promote platelet aggregation and vasoconstriction. Narrowed blood vessels and activated platelets could easily set the stage for a myocardial infarction.

The COX 2-inhibiting drugs are very effective for treating arthritis, and many people derive considerable benefit from their use. If you are currently using a COX 2 inhibitor for arthritis, you should continue to take it and *consult with your doctor regarding the relative risks and benefits of this treatment for you*. The relationship between inflammatory factors and platelet-activating factors is complex. Many new agents under development will attempt to modulate these pathways, but in the treatment of coronary heart disease, plain old aspirin remains the standard for inhibiting platelet aggregation.

Aspirin's efficacy as a treatment of coronary heart disease is well documented. But there is an important difference between its prophylactic use, the prevention of atherosclerosis development, and its use for treating angina symptoms. The largest clinical trial of prophylactic aspirin use was the Physicians Health Study, a prospective, randomized, double-blind, placebo-controlled clinical trial completed in the 1980s. This trial involved 22,000 men. Prophylactic aspirin use reduced the incidence of heart attack by 44 percent. While this result may seem impressive, it is important to recognize that the *absolute reduction* in the incidence of heart attack (that is, the total number of heart attacks prevented) was actually very low. Many people were treated, and some had a very low likelihood of having a heart attack. This study suggested that the greatest benefit of aspirin use occurs in patients who are at high risk of having a heart attack. This seems to be in people over age 50, when the incidence of coronary heart disease is known to increase. The Physicians Health Study involved only men, and it is not certain whether this slight benefit of prophylactic aspirin can be extended to women.

The role of aspirin therapy in the treatment of people with symptomatic coronary heart disease is much clearer than its role in prevention. Anyone who has symptoms of angina or has had a heart attack is known to have coronary heart disease. In 1994, The Antiplatelet Trialists' Collaboration Study pooled the data of numerous clinical trials in what is commonly referred to as a meta-analysis. In this report of 70,000 patients, aspirin treatment was associated with a 25 percent reduction in the incidence of a second heart attack, stroke, or death. Unlike in the Physicians Health Study, the absolute reduction in mortality in this trial was approximately 4 percent. This corresponds to 40 lives saved for every 1,000 patients treated with aspirin, which translates into huge numbers of lives saved among the tens of millions of people with symptomatic atherosclerosis. In the Antiplatelet Trialists' Collaboration, this benefit of aspirin therapy seemed to extend to all people with symptomatic coronary heart disease—both men and women, and people with diabetes. The analysis included other antiplatelet therapies besides aspirin, though aspirin was used in most trials, and the Antiplatelet Trialists' Collaboration confirmed the importance of platelet inhibition in the treatment of coronary heart disease. Aspirin, however, is just one medication that interferes with platelet function. There are other drugs as well.

As noted earlier, aspirin inhibits platelet activation by blocking the actions of the COX enzymes. But blocking this pathway for platelet activation inhibits platelet function by only about 30 percent, because platelets may be activated by several pathways, each with its own set of chemical stimuli. *Adenosine diphosphate* (ADP) is another potent stimulus of platelet aggregation and activation. ADP is present at the site of endothelial damage and is released by activated platelets that are initially drawn to the site. ADP released by activated platelets is an essential component in the self-propagating cascade that leads to the formation of a platelet plug. Blocking ADP limits further platelet activation and aggregation—aggregation that actively contributes to an unstable atherosclerotic plaque. Two drugs, ticlopidine (Ticlid) and clopidogrel (Plavix), are very effective at inhibiting ADP-induced platelet activation. Both are available only by prescription. Of the two, ticlopidine has been associated with significantly more side effects and is less commonly prescribed.

Initially used as a partial anticoagulant for people with coronary stents, clopidogrel is considered by some physicians to be an alternative or an adjunct to aspirin therapy. Clopidogrel seems to be more potent than aspirin in inhibiting platelet function. Whether this action translated into a clinical benefit or increased bleeding risk was unknown until 1996. In that year, the Clopidogrel versus Aspirin in Patients at Risk for Ischemic Events (CAPRIE) trial (a randomized, double-blind, prospective trial) was designed to answer this question. CAPRIE enrolled over 19,000 patients with known coronary heart disease who were randomized to receive either 75 milligrams of clopidogrel or 325 milligrams of aspirin each day. In this study, clopidogrel was marginally better than aspirin in preventing heart attack, stroke, and death (5.3 percent vs. 5.8 percent). This benefit was largely derived by a reduction in the incidence of stroke. The difference was marginal but statistically significant, so CAPRIE has identified clopidogrel as a viable alternative to aspirin in people who are aspirin allergic and require platelet inhibition for the prevention of coronary heart disease.

Considering the role of platelets in coronary heart disease, it makes sense to wonder, if a little platelet inhibition is good, could a lot of platelet inhibition be better? The Clopidogrel in Unstable Angina to Prevent Recurrent Events (CURE) trial was designed to answer this question. In this placebo-controlled trial, over 12,000 highly symptomatic patients randomly received either the combination of clopidogrel plus aspirin (*dual platelet inhibition*) or aspirin alone as part of their treatment for unstable angina. As shown in the results published in 2001, dual platelet inhibition was significantly better than aspirin treatment alone in preventing heart attack, stroke, and death. The benefit of dual platelet inhibition did come at some cost, however. The combination of clopidogrel and aspirin was associated with a higher incidence of a major bleeding episode. Accordingly, the use of dual platelet therapy for the treatment of coronary heart disease is reserved for patients with unstable symptoms or those who are identified as high risk for future cardiac events. Your doctor will help decide which form of platelet inhibition is best for you.

Whether through single therapy or dual therapy, inhibiting platelet function is an important part of coronary heart disease treatment. If you have coronary heart disease, you must inhibit platelets with aspirin or clopidogrel or, sometimes, both. As noted, platelet inhibition is only one part of controlling atherosclerosis. Cholesterol inhibition plays an equally important role.

How Many Ways Can You Lower Cholesterol?

In chapter 2 we explored the pivotal role of LDL cholesterol in the formation of atherosclerotic plaque. The compelling data surrounding

LDL cholesterol and plaque formation leave little room for questioning whether reducing LDL is associated with a reduction in atherosclerotic plaque formation, reduction in progression to a heart attack, and ultimately, an improvement in prognosis. As noted in chapter 4, a family of drugs known as statins are the single most potent agents available for the reduction of LDL cholesterol. The statins listed in chapter 4 are all very effective in reducing LDL.

Over the long term, statins help prevent atherosclerosis, and there is evidence to suggest that they may have an immediate role in the treatment of active, symptomatic coronary heart disease as well. Chapter 3 reviewed data from the REVERSAL trial, in which statin use was associated with a decline in the inflammatory marker hs-CRP. Statin agents also seem to play an important role in reducing arterial wall inflammation and improving the ability of the artery to respond to endogenous vasodilators. This improved vasodilator response helps the coronary arteries respond to the heart's demand for an increase in blood supply. Statins' ability to reduce arterial inflammation and improve endothelial function opens the door for the use of statin agents in acute coronary syndrome. Acute coronary syndrome is unstable angina or angina accompanied by a small rise in cardiac enzymes. Untreated acute coronary syndrome can progress to heart attack.

The Myocardial Ischemia Reduction with Acute Cholesterol Lowering (MIRACL) trial was a prospective, randomized, double-blind, placebo-controlled trial conducted in the late 1990s and designed to test whether early treatment with high doses of statins could reduce the incidence of heart attack or death in people with an acute coronary syndrome. MIRACL showed that high-dose atorvastatin, when started within twenty-four to ninety-six hours of hospital admission for angina or a heart attack, significantly reduced the incidence of repeat heart attack, reduced mortality, and reduced the need for emergency rehospitalization. Unlike the benefits of LDL reduction, the benefits of statin agents did not take years to accrue but were noticed in a matter of days to weeks. MIRACL was the first clinical trial to suggest that these powerful statin agents could be used in ways other than originally intended. Statin agents now play a very important role in all people with coronary heart disease, not only as a way of reducing LDL over the long term but also as a means of preventing recurrent symptoms and reducing death over the short term. The diverse actions of this group of drugs explain why even patients with normal cholesterol levels can benefit from taking a statin. In certain situations, statins can provide benefits independently of their LDL-lowering properties.

Statins are very powerful and useful drugs, but they are not right for everyone. Some people experience side effects with one or even all the statin agents. The most common adverse effect of statin agents is *myopathy*, or muscle weakness. Most clinical trials report an incidence of myopathy ranging from 0.1 to 0.2 percent of all patients treated. This side effect can occur any time between two weeks and two years following the initiation of therapy. The degree of myopathy varies from some muscular soreness to life-threatening destruction of muscle tissue. This latter condition is referred to as *rhabdomyolysis* (rab-dō-mī-äl´-ə-səs) and is the principal reason some statin agents have been withdrawn from the market. Many people are fearful of statin agents because of concern about myopathy. It's important to put this risk into perspective.

The risk of statin-induced complications was brought to the public's attention when cerivastatin was withdrawn from the market because of a risk of fatal rhabdomyolysis that exceeded 3 per 1,000,000 prescriptions. With other statin agents, the average incidence of fatal rhabdomyolysis is less than 1 fatality per 1,000,000 prescriptions (0.0001 percent). A threefold increase in mortality is serious, and removing the drug from the market was the correct action. To put this risk in a somewhat different perspective, however, consider that your risk of being struck by lightning is about 0.00025 percent. This doesn't keep you from going outside, but you do exercise reasonable caution when the risk of a lightning strike is high.

The risk of fatal rhabdomyolysis with statin use is likewise very low, and you should exercise caution when your individual circumstances (such as taking certain medications; see below) may significantly increase this risk. The severity of an individual patient's condition may justify, for the physician and for the patient, an increased risk of rhabdomyolysis or liver inflammation. For most people, the benefits of statin therapy far outweigh the risks of treatment.

While the incidence of statin-related fatal rhabdomyolysis is

0.0001 percent, nonfatal muscle-related symptoms are much more common, affecting between 0.1 and 0.5 percent of people taking statin agents. For some of them, symptoms are severe enough to warrant discontinuing the drug.

Another potential adverse effect of statin agents is liver injury (see table 6.1). When it occurs, the degree of injury is generally mild and is apparent only with blood tests. The incidence of *significant* liver inflammation is quite low, less than 1 percent. There does appear to be a mild dose-dependent increase in the risk of liver inflammation for all statin agents. This risk does not appear to be higher in older people but may be higher in people with certain conditions that affect liver function. Your doctor can help you decide if statin therapy is suitable for you.

Exactly how the statin agents cause muscle or liver damage is not entirely clear. The best available data suggest that toxic levels of statin agents may build up if they are unable to be properly metabolized and subsequently eliminated from the body. The chemical pathway that performs these complex processes resides in the liver and is referred to as the *cytochrome pathway*.

Statin agents are not the only medications that must be modified by the cytochrome pathway prior to elimination. Many medications use this elimination pathway. If a person is taking several of the medications that use this pathway, a logjam of drugs might form in the liver, waiting their turn to be metabolized by the cytochrome system. Due to the delay in being metabolized, some drugs may build up to toxic levels, damaging muscle or liver tissue. The risk of rhabdomyolysis with a statin agent may be increased if you are taking drugs that compete for the same route of elimination.

The list of medications that may increase the risk of rhabdomyolysis is long. The most common are

- fibrates,
- antibiotics of the erythromycin family,
- certain antifungal agents,
- immunosuppressive agents like cyclosporine, and
- some of the medications used to treat HIV infections.

TABLE 6.1 *Risk of Liver Injury with Statins*

	Placebo (%)	Statin 10 mg (%)	Statin 20 mg (%)	Statin 40 mg (%)	Statin 80 mg (%)
Lovastatin	0.1		0.1	0.9	2.3
Simvastatin			0.7	0.9	2.1
Pravastatin	1.3			1.4	
Fluvastatin	0.28		0.2	1.5	2.7
Atorvastatin		0.2	0.2	0.6	2.3
Rosuvastatin		0.0	0.0	0.1	

Source: Data extracted from package inserts and from de Denus et al., "Statins and Liver Toxicity: A Meta Analysis," *Pharmacotherapy* 24, no. 5 (2004): 584–91.

Some statin agents may interfere with the metabolism of Coumadin and thereby increase the risk of bleeding. Statin agents must be prescribed, and their use must be monitored by a physician, usually through routine blood tests once or twice a year. Their considerable benefit to patients with coronary heart disease usually offsets the small risks associated with their use. You should not discontinue using a statin agent without the advice of your physician.

In some people, even the maximum dose of a statin agent does not achieve sufficient reduction in LDL cholesterol. For these people, additional options are available. I want to be clear that I mean *additional*, not *substituted* options. The data supporting the use of statins in coronary heart disease is so compelling that every patient with documented atherosclerosis or significant cardiovascular risk factors should be treated with one. Living with coronary heart disease means that you should be taking a platelet inhibitor and a statin agent, regardless of how well you feel. If *additional* cholesterol-lowering treatment is required, several options are available.

Fibrates are a separate class of lipid-lowering agents. They are sometimes referred to as PPAR ("pee-par") modulators. PPAR modulators work through a complex series of steps that eventually activate the genes responsible for lipid metabolism, inflammation, and even blood clot activation. There are many types of PPAR modulators. Drugs called PPAR gamma modulators (thiazolidinediones) are predominantly used in the treatment of diabetes. There has been some concern that this group of drugs (rosiglitazone, marketed as Avandia) may actually increase the risk of heart attacks. The data are thus far inconclusive, and additional clinical trials addressing this issue are under way. If you are taking a PPAR gamma modulator, you should not stop taking this drug without the advice and agreement of your physician.

The fibrates belong to a different group of PPAR modulators targeting *PPAR alpha*. Working primarily in the liver, fibrates initiate a complex series of actions that alter the relationships among triglycerides, LDL, HDL, and their lipoprotein envelopes. Fibrates' predominant effect is to reduce circulating triglyceride levels. They also appear to have some ability to lower LDL cholesterol as well as produce a modest rise in HDL. Fibrates lower LDL nowhere near as effectively as statin agents. What fibrates do is change the size and density of circulating LDL particles so that they are less atherogenic (less likely to form deposits on arterial walls). Nonetheless, fibrates cannot be considered primary anticholesterol therapy for patients with atherosclerosis. The best use of fibrates seems to be for people with diabetes mellitus or the metabolic syndrome. Here the actions of fibrates may be ideally suited to the situation where the level of circulating triglycerides is high and the level of HDL fairly low. Working primarily in the liver, fibrates need to be taken with caution by patients receiving treatment with a statin agent, because they increase the risk of myopathy and liver injury.

Nicotinic acid, or niacin (vitamin B6), can also affect cholesterol metabolism. It too tends to alter the relative transport of lipids within the liver by favoring the elimination of triglycerides and the formation of HDL. It has only a modest effect on LDL. It cannot be considered a substitute for a statin. Like fibrate agents, niacin's most useful role may be as an adjunct to a statin treatment in people with very low HDL or elevated triglycerides. Like fibrate agents, niacin can increase the risk of myopathy and liver injury when used in combination with statins. As noted in chapter 2, the greatest barrier to niacin use has been the unpleasant flushing that accompanies its treatment. The identification of receptors (in the skin and blood vessels) has opened the door for the creation of niacinlike drugs that do not produce flushing. Clinical trials are under way. Although it is currently available over the counter, niacin should be taken only under the supervision of a physician.

Recall that there are two sources of cholesterol: the measured total cholesterol level is a combination of the *cholesterol that is produced by the liver* and *dietary cholesterol that is absorbed by the intestine*. Eliminating cholesterol from your diet (which is hard to do) and blocking its absorption are potent means of reducing cholesterol. In chapter 4, we discussed the LRC-CPPT, a study that documented the benefit of lowering cholesterol with cholestyramine, which effectively binds dietary cholesterol, preventing its absorption. As noted, cholestyramine is simply too cumbersome to use. Some new drugs appear to be effective in blocking the uptake of dietary cholesterol by the intestine, however.

Ezetimibe (Zetia), unlike cholestyramine, does not bind to dietary cholesterol or bile acids. Rather, ezetimibe seems to work by a unique mechanism that directly alters the lining of the intestine, thus impairing its ability to absorb dietary cholesterol. The primary effect on LDL cholesterol is modest, resulting in an approximate 17 percent reduction. An attractive feature of ezetimibe is that it is very well tolerated. When compared to a placebo, ezetimibe did not have a significantly higher incidence of side effects. As a cholesterol-lowering agent, ezetimibe is pretty good. Unlike statin agents, there is no evidence to suggest that ezetimibe has any effect on plaque inflammation or endothelial function. Also unlike statin agents, there are no compelling long-term mortality data supporting its use as a single agent.

Ezetimibe is not considered initial therapy for people with atherosclerotic disease, nor is it an effective substitute for a statin agent. The greatest advantage of ezetimibe may be in its use as an adjunctive agent to conventional statin therapy. The use of ezetimibe with a statin represents a dual approach to elevated cholesterol, attacking both dietary absorption and hepatic (liver) production. Current evidence suggests that combining ezetimibe with conventional statin therapy will result in an *additional* 25 to 35 percent reduction in LDL cholesterol. This combination therapy does not seem to increase the risk of myopathy or liver injury and appears promising for people with particularly resilient cholesterol levels. The combination of ezetimibe and a low-dose statin is currently available in a single pill marketed as Vytorin (simvastatin and ezetimibe). Aside from convenience, there is nothing unique about this combination pill, and there is nothing to suggest that ezetimibe cannot be combined with other statin agents in the form of separate pills.

People with coronary heart disease require long-term medical therapy. The importance of antiplatelet therapy and anticholesterol therapy in suppressing this disease cannot be overemphasized. These treatments are vital for both the short-term treatment of symptomatic atherosclerosis and the long-term suppression of atherosclerosis. Unfortunately, these treatments are often not enough. People with symptomatic coronary heart disease have a myocardial blood supply that is insufficient to meet the demands of certain activities, and they require additional therapies that will enable the heart to accommodate to the reduced blood supply. Insight into these therapies was gained over a hundred years ago in the munitions factories in Europe.

How Does Nitroglycerin Work?

In the mid-1800s, many people were puzzled by the observation that munitions workers with angina frequently experienced relief of their symptoms while at work and a return of their symptoms when they were at home. Likewise, the incidence of heart attacks that occurred on the weekend seemed disproportionately high. Curiously, for workers with angina, there seemed to be something clinically therapeutic about working in a munitions factory. It was a well-known fact that munitions workers frequently developed flushing and headaches while working with the explosive nitroglycerin. Many workers tolerated this minor annoyance, for the symptoms frequently subsided after they were at work for a few days. These two very disparate, yet significant, observations would serve as a stimulus for much work on the medicinal uses of nitroglycerin.

Nineteenth-century physicians speculated that while at work in the factory, the munitions workers were covered with nitroglycerin, which produced flushing and headaches from vasodilation that was somehow therapeutic for their angina. Over the weekend, the workers' exposure to the nitroglycerin was eliminated, and their blood vessels constricted, often intensely. In workers with coronary heart disease, this overconstriction was detrimental, leading to increased angina and heart attacks. It seemed that, despite the headaches, these workers were more comfortable and even safer while handling explosives at work.

Given the explosive nature of nitroglycerin, the substance obviously could not be studied in humans in any practical way. The inhaled chemical amyl nitrate proved to be a viable alternative for clinical investigation. Subsequent physiological studies revealed that inhaled amyl nitrate had potent effects on the blood vessels, causing them to dilate (vasodilation). As was the case with the munitions workers, flushing and headaches were frequent accompaniments. Amyl nitrate also seemed to relieve the symptoms of angina temporarily. These effects were similar to what was observed in munitions workers handling nitroglycerin.

Recognizing the medicinal possibilities of nitrate-containing compounds opened the door to a new era in the treatment of heart disease. Chemically modified and stable nitroglycerin soon became the staple of treatment for people with angina. It would take another century (and a couple of Nobel prizes) to comprehend how and why this remarkable compound works to relieve angina.

Understanding how nitrates work involved unraveling a seemingly paradoxical observation. For some time, scientists were puzzled by the observation that under some conditions, certain substances could cause a blood vessel to dilate, and yet at other times, the very same substance could cause blood vessel constriction. How could one substance seem to produce opposite results? The answer to this paradox lies in the presence or absence of the vascular endothelium, the thin lining of cells inside every blood vessel in the body.

The endothelium, as we have discussed, is an active barrier that plays an integral part in the regulation of blood vessel diameter. It turns out that the structural integrity of the endothelium determines whether a blood vessel will dilate or constrict in response to a particular chemical stimulus. When the endothelium is intact, some substances produce vasodilation. When the endothelium is damaged (for example, by atherosclerotic plaque), the same substance produces vasoconstriction. These observations raised many questions. How did substances traveling in the bloodstream instruct the blood vessel to dilate or to constrict? How was the message to either dilate or constrict transmitted from the bloodstream to the smooth muscle cells inside the blood vessel wall? As we will discuss, the endothelium is more than a protective barrier; it also acts as a sort of relay station to transmit chemical messages between the bloodstream and the blood vessel wall.

Nitroglycerin may enter the body from various routes. It may be ingested, absorbed through the skin, or injected directly into a vein or an artery. Once in the body, it travels through the bloodstream, bathing the endothelial cells that line the blood vessels. It is then absorbed by the endothelial cells, where it undergoes a biochemical transformation. The exact nature of this biotransformation is not completely understood but the result is that the endothelium cells use this extra source of nitrogen to produce increased levels of nitric oxide (NO) inside the blood vessel wall. (Nitric oxide is not laughing gas, which is nitro*us* oxide, or NO_2.) You may recognize NO as one of the common constituents of air pollution. In the body, however, NO causes no harm. Rather, NO is an essential but short-lived vasodilator. Endothelial-derived NO is the potent vasodilator our body uses to regulate the size of blood vessels. By absorbing some nitroglycerin, we give the body a means of making a little more of the raw materials it needs to manufacture NO. With more nitroglycerin available, more NO is made in the endothelium, resulting in larger blood vessels.

The endothelial lining of the blood vessel is very important in the conversion of the nitroglycerin to NO. The cells of the endothelium serve as factories for the local production of NO. Arteries damaged by the atherosclerotic process have an impaired ability to adjust their size because the NO factories in the endothelial cells are no longer functioning well. The administration of nitroglycerin can give them a much needed boost. Some medications may enhance the synthetic properties of the endothelium. Medications such as statin agents and estrogens can also enhance the endothelium's ability to respond to NO stimulation. While we do not entirely understand this process, we can say that endothelial function can be improved by certain medications.

Nitroglycerin-containing compounds, and nitric oxide in particular, are very important in treating people with symptomatic coronary heart disease. Neither compound actually causes the blood vessels to dilate; rather, both are merely intermediate steps in a chemical cascade that eventually results in vasodilation. The availability of nitroglycerin initiates a chain reaction. The product of this chain reaction is a compound referred to as *cGMP*. It is cGMP, not NO, that signals the smooth muscle cells in the arterial wall to expand. This last step in the chemical cascade is significant because all the nitroglycerin in the world won't work if your body can't make enough cGMP. Likewise, if you have too much cGMP, even a little bit of nitroglycerin can cause an excessive amount of vasodilation.

It is logical to conclude that nitroglycerin prevents angina by dilating the coronary arteries and, in doing so, increasing coronary blood flow, but this is not how nitroglycerin relieves angina. The primary physiological effect of nitroglycerin is an intense *venodilation*. Nitroglycerin preferentially dilates *veins*; although the coronary arteries may dilate, they do so to a much lesser extent than veins elsewhere in the body. Here is what happens. The dilation of the veins in the legs and the abdomen produced by nitroglycerin has the effect of reducing the amount of blood returning to the heart. With less blood returning to the heart, the heart shrinks. Nitroglycerin causes pressure in the heart's chambers to fall abruptly. The decline in blood pressure, in turn, reduces the tension on the heart walls. With less wall tension, the heart consumes less oxygen and the angina goes away. Using nitroglycerin relieves angina, but not by increasing the heart's blood supply. It does so by *reducing the heart's demand for oxygen.* Think of nitroglycerin as a pressure relief valve that can be used when the engine is overworked and hurting. This concept of reducing myocardial oxygen demand rather than increasing myocardial oxygen supply is the cornerstone of the medical treatment of angina. It is a concept that will be used to treat angina again and again.

Nitroglycerin is only one of a family of compounds collectively referred to as *nitrates*. Nitrates were one of the first and continue to be one of the best ways to treat symptomatic angina. But there are some problems with nitrate treatment of angina. Since nitrates work by reducing blood pressure, *if your blood pressure is already low to begin with,* using a nitrate may cause it to become dangerously low. Accordingly, nitrates cannot be used by people with low blood pressure or certain forms of valvular heart disease. Even in a person with normal blood pressure, nitrates may cause lightheadedness if he or she has been standing too long or has not had enough to eat or drink. If you regularly get lightheaded when you use nitrates, you should contact your physician.

Maintaining adequate blood pressure is important when using nitrate-containing compounds. Earlier, I mentioned that it was cGMP that actually signaled the vascular smooth muscle cells to dilate. Think about what might happen if for some reason you had too much cGMP around. Under normal circumstances, cGMP doesn't linger; it is rapidly degraded by other chemical reactions. But several medications may interfere with the degradation of cGMP, and medications that prolong the life of cGMP will prolong vasodilation and make it more intense. In conditions like erectile dysfunction, this type of vascular engorgement is considered a benefit. Sildenafil, vardenafil, and tadalafil (Viagra, Levitra, and Cialis, the medications commonly prescribed for erectile dysfunction, or ED) all interfere with the degradation of cGMP. In the presence of any of these medications, the potency of nitrates is markedly increased. If the nitrates stimulate the production of cGMP, and the ED drugs block the degradation of cGMP, all of a sudden there is a major problem—too much cGMP. The resulting vasodilation can be so intense that a prolonged and unsafe fall in blood pressure may occur.

You cannot use nitrate-containing medications if you regularly use an ED medication. And you cannot use a nitrate-containing medication for up to several days after using a drug for treating erectile dysfunction, depending on the type of ED medication used. For your own safety, if you go to an emergency room because you are having symptoms of chest pain, you must be candid and tell the ER medical staff that you use ED medications.

Too much cGMP is a problem, and so is too little. Too much can cause an excessive vasodilation, and not enough may result in insufficient vasodilation. Remember the munitions workers whose headaches and flushing would go away after a couple of days at work? Prolonged use of nitrates has been associated with *tolerance* of the usual signs of vasodilation. Simply put, the nitrates are no longer working as well. The reasons for this are not entirely clear, but current thinking is that prolonged used of nitrates causes a depletion of cGMP or some of the components required for its synthesis. As a result, nitrate therapy must always be associated with a nitrate-free period, a time during which the body does not see any nitrate-containing compounds. This period of *pharmacological abstinence* enables the body to restore the building blocks required for further cGMP synthesis. The munitions workers, while continuously exposed to nitroglycerin, eventually ran out of building blocks needed to produce vasodilation. Their headaches and flushing then went away. The need to periodically restock our chemical stores of cGMP explains how nitrate-containing medications are currently prescribed.

Nitrates are prescribed in several different preparations. Nearly everyone is familiar with the small nitroglycerin tablet that is placed under the tongue (taken *sublingually*) for the immediate relief of anginal symptoms. This short-acting pill is rapidly dissolved and absorbed into the bloodstream, producing an intense vasodilation within minutes of administration. Unfortunately, the duration of sublingual nitroglycerin action is also very short, lasting only minutes. It's a very good way to relieve symptoms immediately, but this form of nitrate does not provide any extended benefit.

There are several oral preparations of nitrate-containing compounds that have a somewhat longer onset and duration of action. When taken orally, the nitrate must first be absorbed by the intestine and then chemically modified by the liver. Therefore, the potency and duration of action of oral nitrates may vary from person to person. These oral medications are often referred to as isosorbide mononitrate or isosorbide dinitrate. Aside from the route of administration and the duration of action, these medications work just like the old familiar nitroglycerin. These drugs can be difficult to use because the *dose response* (that is, the amount of drug that must be used to produce a vasodilator effect) can vary considerably from one person to the next, and therefore the use of oral nitrates may require frequent adjustment of doses. Some people prefer the oral route of taking nitrates because they don't experience much headache. But the lack of or a mild headache may simply mean that they are not absorbing enough isosorbide or not producing enough nitric oxide to produce any degree of vasodilation.

As seen with the story of the munitions workers, nitroglycerin is well absorbed through the skin. In this route, there is much less variation in the dose needed to produce a clinical effect. Nitroglycerin ointment or paste takes advantage of this fact. For maximal benefit, nitroglycerin ointment generally must be freshly applied to the skin every four to six hours. The frequency of dosing and the mess associated with the use of nitroglycerin ointment can make it inconvenient to use, which is one reason long-acting sustained-release patches containing nitroglycerin have become popular.

One potential problem with sustained-release preparations is that they are so convenient, many patients forget they are wearing one. If they experience sustained delivery of nitroglycerin over several days, they, like the munitions workers, soon can become tolerant of the nitroglycerin. This can usually be avoided by ensuring that a nitrate-free period of six to eight hours occurs each day, usually by removing the nitroglycerin patch at bedtime. It is important to wipe the skin and remove any residual nitroglycerin ointment that may be present.

If you are living with coronary heart disease, you need to know all about nitrate therapy, including what the drug can and cannot do and how it can help and possibly hurt. Nitrate therapy allows patients to live better, have greater exercise capacity, and experience a higher quality of life. Nitroglycerin is a very effective although somewhat cumbersome drug for treating the symptoms of coronary heart disease. While very effective in relieving chest discomfort, nitroglycerin use does not appear to improve survival for patients with symptoms of angina. Nitroglycerin therapy is only one means of reducing myocardial oxygen consumption, however. There are many others drugs that perform this same feat through very different actions.

A Chemical Embargo of the Heart

We've all had that sensation of being scared and feeling our heart race, that sensation that tells the body to get ready for trouble. It is an energized feeling, as if we had just received an injection of high-octane fuel. This reaction is sometimes referred to as the fight-or-flight response. It is a physiological response that is characterized by rapid and vigorous contractions of the heart, increased blood flow to the muscles, and dilation of the pupils. Our body liberates more sugar for a quick burst of energy. In an instant, the body is primed and ready for any intense action that might be required. This response is a remarkable call to arms. How can it happen so fast? How can it all happen at once? Somehow the body must be able to send signals simultaneously to several locations to alert them that it is time to get ready for action.

An elaborate system of chemical signals can fine-tune the output of the body in a manner similar to the fuel injection system in a car. In your car, you step on the gas, inject a little more fuel into the cylinders, and hear the engine rev. In your body, this fuel is *epinephrine* (sometimes called *adrenaline*). With extra epinephrine in the bloodstream, your heart rate increases, the force of cardiac contraction increases, and your blood pressure rises.

The actions of your heart and blood vessels are tightly controlled by a system of chemical signals that instruct them in what to do, literally, from beat to beat. These chemical signals may originate from nerve endings or any of several different sensors that exist throughout the body. Similar to the pony express, these chemical signals are passed along from messenger to messenger until they reach their destination. The instructions may change hands a few times, but ultimately they get to where they are needed, and the appropriate action is taken. Here's how.

Your body is full of chemical sensors that constantly monitor its operating conditions. When one of these types of sensors detects a need for some type of action, it triggers a chemical signal that is released into the bloodstream. This signal is rapidly transported through the bloodstream and ultimately presented to the organ that can provide the help that is needed. In the cardiovascular system, epinephrine and several other similar compounds serve as the chemical signals that help control the speed and vigor of your engine. These chemical signals represent the voice of an elaborate communications network called the *sympathetic and parasympathetic nervous systems*. Understanding how these regulatory systems communicate with the heart will provide another opportunity to see how a very different class of antianginal drugs works.

Thus far, I have portrayed the inside of a normal blood vessel as lined with endothelial cells, forming a smooth pipe. In reality, the endothelial cells are not all that smooth. All the cells in the body look more like fuzz balls than smooth poker chips. Protruding through the surface of every cell in the body are thousands of tiny antennas called *cell surface receptors.* Cell surface receptors monitor the environment outside the cell and control how instructions from outside are communicated to the command centers inside the cell. Like the outstretched hand of the pony express rider, the cell surface receptor extends outside the cell, waiting for the appropriate signal to arrive. When the signal arrives, the receptor rapidly transmits this message to a second messenger inside the cell. Cell surface receptors continuously monitor the outside environment, looking for a unique chemical signal. Much like a lock and key, any given cell surface receptor can bind with one and only one type of chemical signal, and therefore there are unique cell surface receptors for each of the numerous chemical signals that travel through the body. A chemical signal that correctly binds with a receptor is called an *agonist.*

In the cardiovascular system, epinephrine is one of the key agonists. In response to an external threat, our adrenal glands release epinephrine and several other chemical signals into the bloodstream. The epinephrine molecules rapidly travel to the heart, where they bind with a unique cell surface receptor. This union of the proper agonist and the receptor signals the cardiac cells to contract harder and beat faster. Similarly and simultaneously, other epinephrine molecules communicate with the smooth muscle cells in the blood vessel wall, signaling them to dilate. The dilated coronary artery is now ready to accept the increased output from a stimulated heart.

Epinephrine is only one of the cardiac agonists that circulate in the bloodstream. Some may cause the heart to speed up. Others may cause it to slow down. Some may tell the heart to pump harder; others tell it to relax. Depending on the type of cardiac action you require, all you need to do is release the proper type of agonist into the bloodstream. Agonists could be said to come in many different "flavors." Your body knows just what flavor to use to get the job at hand done. Many functions of the heart and blood vessels are controlled by the interactions between these circulating agonists and cell surface receptors. But how do the receptors work? After all, these chemical signals never get to the inside of the heart or blood vessel. Instead, they remain outside, on the cell surface, essentially flipping a chemical switch that lets the cell know that they have arrived and it is time to get to work.

The agonist-receptor union provides the cell with an unequivocal message about what is needed elsewhere in the body. This initial agonist-receptor binding is frequently referred to as the *first message* in the communication chain. A very different *second message* is needed to translate this chemical message from outside the cell into activities that take place inside the cell. When an agonist binds with a cell surface receptor, it changes the shape of the receptor. This conformational change in the receptor is recognized by the chemical machinery inside the cell. The change initiates a cascade of chemical reactions that ultimately leads to the formation of a crucial second messenger. This second messenger travels to the appropriate warehouse inside the cell and fills its order for action. The second messenger is what signals cells to react.

Depending on the type of action required, different types of second messengers are synthesized. For nitroglycerin, the intracellular second messenger is cGMP. The cGMP tells the arterial muscle cells to dilate. For epinephrine and similar chemical signals, the second messenger is a substance called cAMP. As is the case with cGMP, there are substances that can interfere with the degradation of cAMP and cause stimulation of the heart. To a degree, caffeine impairs the degradation of cAMP, which explains why coffee and cola products can make us feel jittery. Medications can also impair the degradation of cAMP. This class of drugs, sometimes referred to as phosphodiesterase inhibitors, are used to treat asthma and congestive heart failure. By mimicking the actions of epinephrine (that is, by increasing levels of cAMP), these medications can worsen angina in patients prone to symptomatic coronary heart disease.

An increased level of cAMP is the heart's signal that it needs a faster heart rate and more vigorous contraction. Receptors that result in an increase in the amount of cAMP are referred to as *adrenergic receptors*. Two types of adrenergic cell surface receptors, called *alpha receptors* and *beta receptors*, are found throughout the cardiovascular system. Stimulation of the alpha receptors on arteries will cause them to constrict; stimulation of the beta receptors will cause arteries to dilate. Alpha receptors tend to be concentrated in vascular smooth muscle, while beta receptors are located in both smooth muscle and cardiac muscle.

By producing predominantly arterial constriction, alpha stimulation will result in elevations in blood pressure. Beta stimulation, while lowering the blood pressure through arterial dilation, also causes the heart to work a lot harder. Beta stimulation does this by dramatically increasing the rate and vigor of contraction. Alpha and beta stimulation increases the heart's work and oxygen consumption. Alpha and beta stimulation is what occurs when we run for a bus, climb a hill, or get overly excited. It is what our body naturally does to rev up the engine to meet the perceived needs of the activity at hand. If your cardiac blood supply is limited by an atherosclerotic coronary artery, the increased oxygen consumption brought about by alpha and beta stimulation can produce angina. Understanding the role of alpha and beta receptors in angina leads directly into the world of cardiac receptor pharmacology.

It seems logical that for every receptor agonist, there should be an antagonist—and there is. But the development of adrenergic receptor antagonists took some doing (and another Nobel Prize). Now a multitude of alpha- and beta-receptor antagonists are available as medications. While there may be minor variations in exactly what they do, they all share the property of blocking the cell surface receptors. Receptor-blocking drugs are molecules that essentially masquerade as agonists. They circulate in the blood and bind with the cell surface receptors without sending the second message. These disguised agonists bind with the cell surface receptors by essentially wrapping them in a shroud that prevents the receptor from interacting with the true agonist that circulates in the body. The development of drugs that can effectively block cell surface receptors is one of the great medical breakthroughs of the twentieth century. Their importance in the treatment of heart disease cannot be overstated.

Receptor-blocking drugs can be very specific. Some are directed at blocking the alpha receptors, some the beta receptors. And some of these drugs block both types of receptors. Let's think about what this means in physiological terms. If alpha stimulation causes blood vessel constriction, alpha-receptor blockade will prevent constriction and result in some vasodilation, lowering blood pressure. If beta stimulation causes an increase in heart rate and an increase in force of cardiac contraction, beta-receptor blockade will prevent any increase in heart rate and limit the vigor of cardiac contraction.

This type of "pharmacological restraint" can be clinically beneficial to patients who have a cardiac blood supply that is limited by an atherosclerotic coronary artery. In this setting, alpha- and beta-blocking drugs function by keeping the heart from entering the "red zone." They keep the blood pressure low and prevent it from rising with exercise. They also keep the heart rate low and prevent it from rising with exercise. In most cases, these pharmacological restraints will prevent myocardial oxygen demand from exceeding the oxygen supply during exercise. The *functional* result is that exercise capacity is often increased. The *clinical* result is that angina will be prevented or delayed.

Beta-Blocking Drugs

Because beta stimulation contributes greatly to myocardial oxygen consumption, beta-blocking drugs are among the most commonly prescribed antianginal agents. The evidence supporting their use in patients with angina is longstanding and substantial. These drugs have been available for use by patients for over thirty years. They are among the most thoroughly tested drugs prescribed today.

Table 6.2 lists the currently available beta-blocking drugs. All are very effective in blocking the beta receptor. Some selectively block subtypes of the beta receptors. Others, to a varying degree, also block the alpha receptor. You doctor can decide which type of beta-receptor-blocking agent is best for your condition.

Because they directly target the cause of anginal symptoms—a myocardial oxygen demand that exceeds the myocardial oxygen supply—beta-blocking drugs are frequently used as a first-line agent for the treatment of angina. Beta blockade can have a dramatic effect on patients with symptomatic coronary heart disease. In a 1976 study, patients treated with the beta-blocking drug propranolol saw a 50 percent reduction in the number of angina episodes and in the need for sublingual nitroglycerin use. This is a dramatic improvement in

TABLE 6.2   *Commonly Prescribed Beta-Blocking Drugs*

Brand Name	Generic Name	Generic Available?
Blocadren	timolol	Yes
Coreg	carvedilol	Yes
Corgard	nadalol	Yes
Inderal	propranolol	Yes
Kerlone	betaxolol	Yes
Levatol	penbutolol	No
Normodyne	labetalol	Yes
Sectral	acebutolol	Yes
Tenormin	atenolol	Yes
Toprol and Lopressor	metoprolol	Yes
Visken	pindolol	Yes
Zebeta	bisoprolol	Yes

lifestyle for patients with symptomatic disease. And, unlike the situation with long-acting nitrates, there was no apparent patient resistance or tolerance to beta blockade. Patients in this study experienced a sustained clinical benefit with beta blockade for up to eight years. These findings can be replicated with virtually any beta-blocking drug. Beta-blocking drugs are very effective antianginal medications, and their efficacy has been repeatedly confirmed in numerous clinical trials.

In addition to preventing the symptoms of angina, beta blockers seem able to do much more. Giving beta-blocking drugs immediately to a person who is experiencing an acute heart attack has been shown to significantly reduce mortality. In people who have already had a heart attack, long-term treatment with beta blockade seems to reduce the risk of a second heart attack and the incidence of sudden death. This outcome is in sharp contrast to nitrate therapy, which appears only to reduce frequency and intensity of angina symptoms without any mortality benefit.

Figure 6.1 graphically depicts the beneficial impact of long-term treatment with propranolol, a beta-blockade medication. The Beta Blocker Heart Attack Trial (BHAT), a prospective, randomized, double-blind, placebo-controlled trial conducted about thirty years ago, evaluated the long-term use of beta blockade in 3,837 patients who had sustained a recent heart attack. The BHAT trial was stopped nine

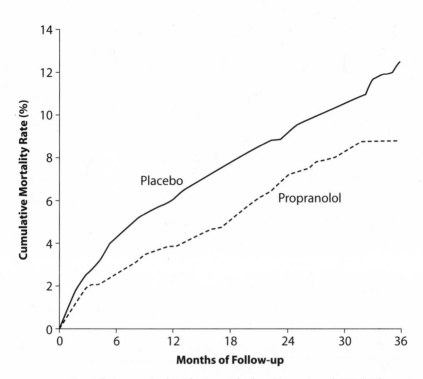

FIGURE 6.1. Cumulative survival in the Beta Blocker Heart Attack Trial. The beneficial impact of the use of beta-blocking drugs following an acute myocardial infarction is illustrated here. The chart underscores the significant reduction in mortality associated with the use of propranolol and shows that this mortality benefit is not accrued until after six months of treatment. (From "A Randomized Trial of Propranolol in Patients with Acute Myocardial Infarction. II. Morbidity Results," *Journal of the American Medical Association* 250 (1983): 2814–19.)

months ahead of schedule when the Data and Safety Monitoring Board recognized the favorable impact of beta-blocking therapy. On average, treatment with beta blockade resulted in a 23 percent reduction in mortality. This mortality benefit, largely brought about by a reduction in the incidence of sudden cardiac death, was apparent soon after the start of the drug and was sustained for many years thereafter.

BHAT showed that in addition to reducing the incidence of death, beta-blocking therapy was associated with a significant reduction in the incidence of nonfatal *repeat* heart attack. The results of BHAT have been confirmed by several other studies involving other beta-blocking agents. The benefit of beta blockade seems to be a class effect and not restricted to one type of beta-blocking drugs. They all seem to work, and they work wonders. Their use has become the standard of care for patients with symptomatic coronary heart disease.

All people with symptomatic coronary heart disease should be treated with a beta-blocking agent unless this treatment is contraindicated. What about side effects? Unfortunately, the "pharmacological restraint" provided by beta blockade may cause some patients to feel tired or to become easily fatigued. By blocking only the beta receptor, these agents may facilitate excessive alpha-receptor stimulation. The unopposed vasoconstriction can lead to a reduction in blood flow to the hands and feet, causing some people to suffer cold extremities. In most cases, these inconveniences are far outweighed by the reduction in angina and the mortality benefit.

Beta-blocking drugs should not be taken by people with medical conditions such as an excessively slow heart rate, certain electrical disorders of the heart, or decompensated congestive heart failure. The loss of beta stimulation (produced by beta blockade) may significantly worsen these conditions. Similarly, some people with asthma or emphysema may rely on beta stimulation or drugs that produce beta stimulation. Beta blockade may actually worsen their condition. Beta-blocking drugs may also interact with other drugs that affect the heart rate and vigor of cardiac contraction. Your doctor will assess the risks and benefits of beta-blocking therapy with you.

Alpha-Blocking Drugs

The story behind alpha-receptor-blocking agents is somewhat different. While present in cardiac tissue, alpha receptors are found in much greater numbers in arterial smooth muscle. Because alpha stimulation results primarily in arterial constriction, the primary effect of alpha-receptor blockade is arterial dilation. Accordingly, until recently alpha-receptor-blocking agents have been predominantly used to treat high blood pressure. You may recognize clonidine (Catapres) and prazosin (Minipress) as two of the more popular alpha-blocking agents. Given their potency and side effects, they are not usually used as first-line drugs for the treatment of hypertension. They are, however, frequently used in conjunction with other medications in treating difficult-to-control hypertension.

Alpha adrenergic receptors can be found in the smooth muscle of the bladder wall as well as in the prostate gland in men. Thus, in recent years, alpha-receptor-blocking agents have found a new role in the combined treatment of hypertension and urinary frequency in men with prostate enlargement. Doxazosin (Cardura), tamsulosin (Flomax), and terazosin (Hytrin) are all very effective in treating urinary frequency caused by an enlarged prostate gland.

These drugs, even when used to improve urinary symptoms, are also potent antihypertensive agents. When used for an extended period, they do a very good job of blocking alpha receptors from any form of alpha stimulation. If any of these medications is abruptly stopped, the "naive" alpha receptors can be very sensitive to any circulating alpha agonists, and this may cause an intense vasoconstriction and a dangerous elevation in blood pressure. If you are taking an alpha-blocking agent for any reason, you should never stop taking it without the advice of your physician. *Rebound hypertension* is only one of the possible adverse effects of alpha-blocking drugs. Unfortunately, there are several others: alpha-blocking drugs have some potent effects, and not everyone can tolerate them. With the alpha receptors blocked, fine control of the arterial system is lost. As a result, some people may experience a significant fall in blood pressure when arising from a seated or lying position. In most people, this tendency to become light headed can generally be overcome by arising slowly and staying well hydrated. The tendency to develop low blood pressure when standing is referred to as *orthostatic hypotension*. It frequently limits the use of alpha-blocking agents in older people and in people with diabetes.

Combining Alpha and Beta Blockers

Perhaps the most exciting development in alpha- and beta-receptor pharmacology is the concept of developing drugs with dual actions. This might include combing alpha- and beta-receptor-blocking properties in a single drug or using a drug with both agonist and antagonist properties. These types of agents may be of particular benefit in people with congestive heart failure who seem to have defective alpha and beta cell surface receptors. In people with congestive heart failure, the heart neither contracts vigorously nor responds well to alpha and beta stimulation. Cell surface receptors appear to have worn out over time. Clinical evidence points to the possibility of altering the nature of cell surface receptors. Consider the following.

In chapter 3, congestive heart failure was identified as one of the consequences of a heart attack. Congestive heart failure is caused by a decline in pump function related to an abnormal thickening and enlargement of the heart. When congestive heart failure occurs, the body sends out several chemical signals calling for more vigorous contractions and a faster heart rate. The body responds by flooding the bloodstream with excessive amounts of alpha and beta agonists. Bombarded with an excessive amount of alpha and beta stimulation, the cell surface receptors eventually become unresponsive, and cardiac function continues to deteriorate. (Medically speaking, the unresponsive receptors have become *down regulated,* but one can think of them as just becoming disinterested.)

Prolonged blockade of the dysfunctional receptors with alpha- and beta-receptor-blocking agents stimulates the emergence of new cell surface receptors. The new (and naive) cell surface receptors work very well. These receptors are not fatigued, and they avidly bind any circulating agonists, resulting in significant improvement in ventricular function, improvement in symptoms, and a favorable outcome. The use of low doses of alpha- and beta-blocking agents seems to encourage the elimination of fatigued adrenergic receptors and facilitate the emergence of newer and healthier ones.

The CAPRICORN study is one of several clinical trials that have verified this concept. At the time of the study, about a decade ago, carvedilol (Coreg) was a relatively new agent; it has some alpha-blocking properties but it predominantly has beta-blocking properties. CAPRICORN showed that patients with congestive heart failure related to a prior myocardial infarction had a significant reduction in mortality when treated with carvedilol for six months. This improvement in survival was related to a demonstrable reduction in cardiac size and a significant improvement in contractile function. These beneficial effects of carvedilol treatment were additive to the benefits conferred by standard medical therapy.

Understanding the role of alpha and beta cell surface receptors is a breakthrough for modern cardiovascular medicine. Drugs that were once thought to cause congestive heart failure (alpha- and beta-blocking agents) could now be used to treat it. In the CAPRICORN trial, use of these drugs prevented some of the adverse cardiac remodeling that was described in chapter 3, and in doing so, improved prognosis. There is legitimate debate about whether the benefits observed in CAPRICORN are unique to carvedilol or whether they represent a class effect common to all alpha- and beta-blocking agents. Additional clinical trials are needed to settle this and other important questions regarding the role of these medications in treating coronary heart disease. For now, unless there is a very good reason not to, living with coronary heart disease will mean taking some type of adrenergic-blocking agent. For many people this means the addition of a beta-blocking agent to their growing list of drugs, including platelet inhibitors, statin agents, and a nitrate.

Using a beta-blocking drug is only one way of decreasing the heart's oxygen consumption. Other drugs perform similar actions, such as a class of antianginal drugs called calcium channel blockers. Before understanding them, we must expand our concept of the cell wall and how it interacts with the external environment. Every cell is surrounded by a protective barrier that insulates the inner machinery of the cell from the external environment. We have seen how molecules like nitroglycerin can penetrate this barrier and initiate chemical reactions inside a living cell, and how cell surface receptors stand on guard, monitoring the external environment and passing messages on to the cell's inner workings. There is a third route of entry that allows certain molecules to slip through the cell membrane via a special passage called an *ion channel*.

The Role of Calcium-Channel-Blocking Agents

The cell membrane is crucial in maintaining the balance of sodium, potassium, and calcium inside every cell. For every single beat of the heart, molecules of these chemicals must flow in and out of the cell very quickly. Called *ionic currents,* these flows of molecules occur in fractions of a second and do so via "trap doors" in the cell membrane called ion channels. Much like portholes on a submarine, when one of these channels is opened, ions will flow in or out of the cell. The cell membrane is dotted with ion channels for sodium, potassium, and calcium. For the purposes of treating symptomatic coronary heart disease, the calcium channels are the most important.

For muscle to contract, the concentration of calcium inside the cell must increase. With each beat, the calcium channels on the cell surface membrane open, allowing a rapid flux of calcium into the cell. This high intracellular calcium triggers a contraction of the cardiac cell. When all the heart's cells contract in unison, the muscle shortens and the heart pumps. Simply put, the more calcium inside each cell, the more vigorous the contraction of the heart. We can treat angina by impairing the entry of calcium into cardiac muscle cells, which reduces the heart's oxygen consumption. Impairing the entry of calcium into arterial smooth muscle also causes the muscle cells to dilate.

Being able to block the cell membrane's calcium channel heralded a new era in the treatment of angina. Calcium-channel-blocking agents are another useful therapy in the treatment of atherosclerosis. There are several different calcium-channel-blocking drugs, each varying slightly in the role it plays in maintaining calcium channel balance inside and outside the cell. To some extent, however, they all share common properties: they blunt the vigor of cardiac contraction, lower blood pressure, and slow the heart rate. By regulating the factors that determine myocardial oxygen demand, they are all very effective in relieving the symptoms of angina.

The data supporting the use of channel-blocking drugs in treating chronic stable angina are strong. Like beta-blocking drugs, calcium-channel-blocking drugs have stood the test of time. Some have been available for over twenty-five years. Table 6.3 lists the commonly available calcium-channel-blocking drugs. The three separate categories are primarily based on the chemical structure of the drugs, but the groups do have some significant differences in their physiological actions.

The dihydropyridine class is the largest and most commonly pre-

TABLE 6.3 Calcium-Channel-Blocking Drugs

Dihydropyridine Class		Phenylalkylamine Class		Benzothiazipines Class	
Adalat	nifedipine	Calan	verapamil	Cardizem	diltiazem
Procardia	nifedipine	Isoptin	verapamil	Tiazac	diltiazem
Cardene	nicardipine				
Cardene SR	nicardipine				
Cardif	nitrendipine				
Nitrepin	nitrendipine				
Nomotop	nimodipine				
Norvasc	amlodipine				
Plendil	felodipine				
Sular	nisoldipine				

scribed. These calcium-channel-blocking drugs exert their greatest effect on the calcium channels in vascular smooth muscle. They produce a rather significant arterial vasodilation that tends to lower blood pressure. This arterial vasodilation is not limited to the systemic arteries, however—the coronary arteries dilate as well. Calcium-channel-blocking drugs belonging to the dihydropyridine group have been shown to be particularly useful in people whose conditions include a strong component of coronary spasm. As noted in chapter 5, the clinical significance of a coronary stenosis is related to the combined degree of fixed coronary obstruction (due to atherosclerotic plaque) and dynamic obstruction (due to coronary spasm). By preventing coronary spasm, these calcium-channel-blocking drugs may decrease the severity of a coronary stenosis and increase coronary blood flow. Unfortunately, this ability to produce an arterial vasodilation can also produce facial flushing, salt and water retention (which people usually notice as swelling of the feet in the late afternoon), and a moderate *increase* in heart rate. These well-recognized side effects have limited the usefulness of these drugs for some people. To some degree, these side effects have been reduced by using long-acting preparations, which facilitate a lesser but more prolonged vasodilation. In some instances, these side effects can be circumvented by using the drugs in conjunction with another medication, usually a beta-blocking agent or a diuretic. Because of the side effects, dihydropyridine calcium-blocking drugs are usually reserved as a third-line agent to treat resilient angina.

The phenylalkylamine group of calcium-channel-blocking drugs is quite different. This group of drugs primarily blocks the calcium channels present in cardiac tissue. As a result, the drugs markedly reduce the contractile ability of the heart and have less effect on the arterial smooth muscle lining blood vessels. This reduction in cardiac contractility reduces the amount of work the heart performs with each beat. Working less, the heart consumes less oxygen, and the imbalance between oxygen demand and supply that characterizes angina is resolved. This cardiac suppressant feature can be useful to treat angina *only if you have a very strong heart.* This group of drugs can take the horsepower out of your heart in a hurry. If your heart muscle is already weak, this group of drugs can cause your ventricular function to deteriorate further, producing symptoms of congestive heart failure. These drugs also have potent effects on the heart's electrical system, causing the heart to slow.

The phenylalkylamine group of calcium-channel-blocking drugs can interact with several common cardiac medications like digoxin or amiodarone to produce a significant and potentially dangerous decline in heart rate. When using these drugs, you must be closely monitored by your doctor. For this reason and because of the risks described above, these drugs are seldom used as antianginal agents. Phenylalkylamine drugs are most commonly used in people with angina who have very strong hearts and who cannot take a beta blocker because of asthma or side effects.

The benzothiazipines group, like the phenylalkylamine group, blocks calcium channels in cardiac muscle but to a lesser degree. Like the dihydropyridine group, benzothiazipines produce some arterial vasodilation and can lower blood pressure, but again, they do so to a lesser degree. The benzothiazipine drugs are thought of as "kinder and gentler" calcium-channel-blocking agents. Some caution needs to be exercised with their use, however, because these drugs also interact with the heart's electrical system and can slow the heart rate. Nonetheless, they are very effective in relieving the symptoms of angina by effectively reducing heart rate, blood pressure, and contractility. Among all calcium-channel-blocking agents, drugs from this group may have some role as standalone antianginal agents. They are generally well tolerated.

Nitrates, beta-blocking drugs, and calcium-channel-blocking drugs are all similar in that they reduce myocardial oxygen consumption by altering one or more of the physiological determinants of myocardial oxygen demand: heart rate, blood pressure, or cardiac contractility. Another potential way to treat angina would be to alter the way the heart uses energy. A *metabolic modulator* would represent a new class of antianginal drugs. Under normal conditions, the heart muscle uses large, complicated molecules called free fatty acids as the primary source of energy. Glucose, while a more efficient energy source, is used less often. A drug that could shift the cardiac metabolism from free fatty acids to glucose use would render the heart more efficient and thus less vulnerable to angina.

Metabolic Modulators

Trimetazidine is considered to be a cardiac metabolic modulator. In laboratory studies, trimetazidine has been shown to shift cardiac metabolism toward more efficient glucose use. In limited clinical trials in Europe, trimetazidine has been shown to be more effective than placebo for the treatment of angina. When compared to nitrates or beta-blocking agents, trimetazidine was at least as effective in reducing symptoms and improving exercise capacity. But unlike these drugs, trimetazidine was not associated with any alteration in heart rate or blood pressure. It did not appear to target the usual determinants of myocardial oxygen consumption. The antianginal effects of trimetazidine appear to be solely mediated by an alteration in cardiac metabolism. The ultimate role of trimetazidine for the treatment of angina is not clear. Much about its action is unknown. Additional large prospective, randomized clinical trials will be required before it will be available for use in the United States.

Like trimetazidine, ranolazine (Ranexa) was initially thought to favorably alter cardiac metabolism. Recent studies suggest that this may not be the case. At the usual dose, ranolazine's effects on free fatty acid metabolism are minor. Ranolazine exerts its primary actions on intracellular sodium and calcium metabolism. It seems to limit the amount of calcium that enters the cell and that makes it vulnerable to ischemic injury. Exactly how ranolazine reduces the incidence of angina remains unclear. In several large prospective clinical trials, ranolazine was shown to be effective in the treatment of angina. Compared to a placebo, ranolazine was more effective in improving exercise capacity and in reducing the frequency of anginal attacks.

We do not yet know how ranolazine can be used in the treatment of angina. It has potent effects on the heart's electrical system, and patients taking the medication must be closely monitored with scheduled electrocardiograms. It also has the potential to interact with numerous medications, including digoxin, certain calcium-channel-blocking agents, and some antibiotics. Ranolazine may compete with some statin agents for clearance by the liver, though an increased risk of liver or muscle damage has not been reported. While treatment with ranolazine increases the complexity of medical care, it is another choice for physicians and patients in treating angina.

Blocking the Actions of Angiotensin II

Hypertension is a well-established risk factor for coronary heart disease. As noted in chapter 5, maintaining a healthy blood pressure helps prevent the formation of atherosclerosis and helps prevent its progression in people who already have coronary heart disease. Understanding how the body controls blood pressure provides insights into the available therapeutic options. It may come as a surprise that the key to understanding blood pressure control begins deep within the kidney.

Most people know that the kidney's primary function is to filter blood. Twenty-four hours a day, seven days a week, 365 days a year, the kidneys silently and efficiently eliminate blood-borne toxins that accumulate as byproducts of the body's normal metabolic function. For optimal health, the kidney must closely monitor and regulate this filtration process. Much like a chef sampling an assembly line of baked goods, the kidneys continuously monitor the blood flow and composition, adding a little bit of this, removing a little bit of that to ensure optimal function. Like any good assembly line, the kidneys must maintain a steady flow of blood through their filters. If the blood pressure falls too low, the kidneys can act to increase the blood pressure to their filters. Likewise, if the blood pressure is too high, the kidney can act to lower the filtration pressure. The kidneys are active organs that synthesize various hormones and therefore play an important role in the control of blood pressure. As a modulator of blood pressure, the kidneys are a link between hypertension and the development of heart disease.

The kidney's filter is a microscopic coil of blood vessels called a *glomerulus* (glō-mer´-yə-ləs). There are literally millions of glomeruli throughout the kidneys. The flow into and out of each glomerulus is closely monitored and controlled by the kidney, which adjusts the pressure of the blood that is being filtered. Adjacent to the glomerulus is a dense layer of cells that sense the blood pressure. This pressure-sensitive layer of cells contains a special group of cells referred to as the *juxta glomerular* (JG) apparatus. The kidney's JG cells begin the series of chemical messages that control blood pressure.

The JG cells are packed with tiny granules of a hormone called *renin.* In response to a fall in blood pressure, renin is released into the bloodstream and serves as a chemical smoke signal that tells the body that more blood pressure is needed. The renin signal circulates throughout the body, activating a hormone called angiotensin II. This activation involves several steps, as depicted in figure 6.2. Angiotensin II then binds with a specific receptor found on all blood vessels throughout the body. The stimulated angiotensin II receptor induces the blood vessels to constrict. The resultant vasoconstriction produces a prompt rise in blood pressure.

While the elevation in blood pressure induced by angiotensin II may initially be beneficial, stimulation of the angiotensin II receptors has other properties that, over the long term, may be harmful. These include stimulation of cardiac muscle replication, development of endothelial dysfunction, and ultimately cell death. You will recognize these as ingredients essential to the development of atherosclerosis. Angiotensin II seems to accelerate the development of atherosclerosis. In light of all these deleterious actions, it makes sense that blocking the actions of angiotensin II would have a beneficial effect in people with coronary heart disease.

Referring to figure 6.2, we can see that there are several ways to reduce the activity of angiotensin II. Angiotensin II is formed with the assistance of an enzyme aptly called *angiotensin-converting enzyme*

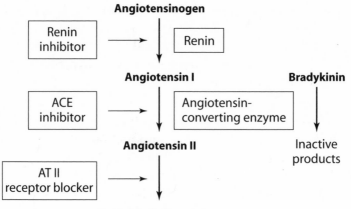

Angiotensinogen

| Renin inhibitor | → | Renin |

Angiotensin I   **Bradykinin**

| ACE inhibitor | → | Angiotensin-converting enzyme |

Angiotensin II   Inactive products

| AT II receptor blocker | → |

Angiotensin II receptors

FIGURE 6.2. The renin angiotensin cascade. Everyone has circulating angio-tensinogen in their blood. When renin is released from the kidney, it facilitates the production of angiotensin I, which is later converted to angiotensin II (AT II) by an enzyme. Angiotensin II stimulates the AT II receptors that are located on blood vessels. This causes them to constrict, resulting in a rise in blood pressure. This diagram depicts the numerous sites where drugs can intervene to prevent the vasoconstriction produced by stimulation of the AT II receptors. There are new drugs available that block the action of renin, angiotensin-converting enzyme, or the AT II receptor itself.

(ACE). Inhibiting the activity of ACE prevents the formation of angiotensin II and prevents many of its actions. Drugs referred to as ACE inhibitors have emerged as some of the most beneficial treatments for people with heart disease. The currently available ACE inhibitors are listed in table 6.4.

Another way to prevent the action of angiotensin II is to block its activity at the level of the angiotensin receptor. A group of drugs called *angiotensin-receptor-blocking agents* (ARB) are also listed in table 6.4. Both ACE inhibitors and ARB agents are very effective in treating hypertension. Given their effects on smooth muscle and endothelial functions, they have emerged as important drugs in the acute and long-term treatment of patients with coronary heart disease.

In the Heart Outcomes Prevention Evaluation (HOPE) trial of the 1990s, over 9,000 patients were prospectively randomized to receive either the ACE inhibitor ramipril or a placebo. To be accepted into

TABLE 6.4   *ACE Inhibitors and ARB Drugs*

Brand Name	Generic Name
Angiotensin-Converting Enzyme Inhibitors	
Lotensin	benazepril
Capoten	captopril
Vasotec	enalapril
Monopril	fosinopril
Prinivil, Zestril	lisinopril
Univasc	moexipril
Aceon	perindopril
Accupril	quinapril
Altace	ramipril
Mavik	trandolapril
Angiotensin-Receptor-Blocking Agents	
Atacand	candesartan
Teveten	eprosartan
Avapro	irbesartan
Cozaar	losartan
Benicar	olmesartan
Micardis	telmisartan
Diovan	valsartan

the study, patients had to be at high risk for cardiovascular disease. Over half the patients in each group had sustained a prior heart attack. A significant number of patients in each group had hypertension, diabetes, or an adverse cholesterol profile. All the patients enrolled in this trial were truly at high risk for the development of coronary heart disease. After five years of treatment, the difference in the incidence of adverse outcome between treatment groups was striking.

After five years of treatment, the ramipril-treated group had a significantly lower incidence of death, cardiac arrest, heart attack, congestive heart failure, stroke, or need for a coronary revascularization procedure. In this high-risk patient population, the use of an ACE inhibitor provided significant protection against adverse events. This effect was even more dramatic in certain very high-risk groups. Further, in this trial, 3,577 people had diabetes, 1,135 of whom had no clinical evidence of cardiovascular disease at the time of their enrollment. In this subgroup of patients, ramipril treatment significantly reduced the chance of developing cardiovascular disease (18.7 percent for placebo vs. 10.2 percent for ramipril). It is important to emphasize that this benefit was accrued in addition to the usual treatment with cholesterol-lowing agents, platelet inhibitors, and beta-blocking drugs. The results of HOPE have been replicated by other studies using different ACE inhibitors and underscore the protective value of angiotensin inhibition.

Inhibition of the renin angiotensin system may have other important implications for people who have had a heart attack. In chapter 3, the concept of cardiac remodeling was introduced. Recall that following a heart attack, the development of scar tissue and subsequent expansion of the scarred area sets the stage for later complications. This adverse cardiac remodeling is associated with an increased likelihood of death due to a higher incidence of congestive heart failure, fatal arrhythmias, or stroke. In people who have sustained an ST-elevation myocardial infarction (STEMI), early treatment with ACE inhibitors has been shown to reduce mortality. This benefit is directly attributable to a reduction in the extent of infarct expansion and resulting preservation of cardiac size and function.

Numerous studies have now shown that treatment with an ACE inhibitor following a heart attack is beneficial. Using these inhibitors has become standard practice in treating people who have had a heart attack. We have discussed other ways to block the adverse effects of angiotensin. An ACE inhibitor is the most common way, and most clinical trials examining this question have used one of these drugs. The effects of angiotensin can also be blocked at the receptor level, however. Relatively few clinical trials have examined the effectiveness of ARB agents following an acute myocardial infarction. In the studies that are available, the data suggest that ARBs are neither better nor worse than ACE inhibitors. Both drugs save lives. Angiotensin-receptor-blocking agents may have a unique role in treating people who cannot tolerate ACE inhibitors due to side effects.

Referring to figure 6.2, note that the angiotensin-converting enzyme also facilitates the degradation of a group of compounds referred to as *bradykinins*. In the setting of ACE inhibition, bradykinins may accumulate, producing a persistent nonproductive cough. Up to 20 percent of people taking an ACE inhibitor develop a persistent cough, and such a cough is the most common reason for discontinuing the drug. The ARB agents can circumvent the accumulation of brady-kinins and still block the effects of angiotensin II at the local receptor level. ARB agents do not produce cough but do produce other side effects.

Some people cannot take either an ACE inhibitor or an ARB agent. Both drugs may worsen kidney function in people with under-lying kidney dysfunction, for example. In fact, anyone taking these medications must have their kidney function and serum potassium level closely monitored with blood tests. There is also some sugges-tion that taking nonsteroidal anti-inflammatory drugs (NSAIDs) with ACE inhibitors or ARBs may not only limit the effectiveness of ACE inhibitors and ARBs but also increase the risk of kidney dysfunction. If you are taking either of these drugs, you should not take other medications, including NSAIDs, without the advice and supervision of your doctor.

Inhibiting the effects of the renin angiotensin system is a very important part of the treatment of cardiovascular disease. There will soon be other medications that are able to interact with this system. Inhibition of plasma renin has always been an attractive target, but developing drugs to do this has been challenging. Aliskiren (Tekturna) is an oral renin inhibitor that has recently been approved by the U.S. Food and Drug Administration for the treatment of hypertension. It promises to have many of the beneficial effects associated with inhibi-tion of the renin angiotensin system. Its exact role in treating patients with coronary heart disease still needs to be determined.

The medical treatment of symptomatic atherosclerosis is com-plex. A multipronged approach is the standard of care, with medica-tions designed to prevent the formation of clots, improve endothelial function, and reduce the heart's myocardial oxygen consumption. Successfully treating this last element and quieting the factors that produce angina frequently requires two or even three different medi-cations. James left his doctor's office with a bag full of medications and prescriptions—and he needed every one of them. While the cost and complexity of these medications can be overwhelming, their im-portance in treating coronary heart disease cannot be denied.

There are many choices for the medical treatment of coronary artery disease. The marketing of these drugs now extends past the literature intended for physicians and can be seen in advertisements in newspapers, popular magazines, and television. While these advertisements may be of value in raising public awareness about the various treatment options, keep in mind that the appropriateness of any drug varies from patient to patient. Working together, you and your doctor can choose the treatment that is best for you. Learning to live with coronary artery disease means knowing not only what these drugs are but how they are likely to affect your condition. With your understanding of coronary artery disease, you are in a better position to ask knowledgeable questions about any prescribed treatment.

The treatments discussed thus far have largely focused on medications to enable the heart to accommodate to the reduction in coronary blood flow that is a consequence of atherosclerosis. There are other therapeutic options available. Atherosclerosis, after all, is an obstructive disorder. The pipes supplying the heart with blood have become blocked, and so it might make sense to consider treatments that might relieve the coronary obstructions and directly improve the myocardial blood supply. James, like many patients, was reluctant to consider invasive treatments. But living with coronary heart disease also involves understanding the role of invasive options as well as medications. It's time to consider these as well.

SEVEN

When Does Balloon Surgery Help?

James was reluctant to take so many medications. The prospect of keeping track of all those pills and paying for them was overwhelming. His doctor told him that the best way to treat his condition was to provide a new blood supply to the heart, a *myocardial revascularization.* James had heard that many types of coronary artery blockages can be fixed with some sort of a balloon surgery. Like many patients, he wanted to know how the procedure worked, whether he was a candidate, whether it was dangerous, and whether the results lasted. In this chapter, we will explore all these topics.

To find out whether a patient is a candidate for the surgery, many doctors recommend a cardiac catheterization. James had the catheterization and he did just fine, but much to his surprise, his doctors decided to admit him to the hospital for observation. James and his family were understandably concerned. The test was originally scheduled to be an outpatient procedure. Now he was a patient in the hospital, and there was talk of open-heart surgery. How could all this be happening so fast? Why were the doctors considering surgery rather than fixing his blockages with a balloon procedure?

The answer to James's question lies in what the coronary angiogram identified about his atherosclerotic disease. During the cardiac catheterization, the doctors performed a coronary angiogram to visualize the quantity and quality of the atherosclerotic narrowings. James's coronary angiogram looked much like figure 5.4b. Several features of his angiogram placed James in an unfavorable prognostic category. He needed urgent hospitalization and medical stabilization before there could be any consideration of how the blood supply to his heart could be improved.

As noted in chapter 5, a coronary angiogram provides an anatomical map of the location and nature of the coronary arterial narrowings. It tells us how many coronary arteries are narrowed, where in the blood vessel the narrowings are located, whether the narrowings are short or long, whether the narrowings are calcified or not, and whether there is evidence of thrombus within the blood vessel. James's angiogram revealed sequential 95 percent narrowings at the origin of his left anterior descending coronary artery (LAD). There was also a large filling defect within the coronary artery representing a thrombus that was located next to one of the narrowings, a defect that threatened to occlude the artery completely at a moment's notice. Additional narrowings of 70 to 80 percent diameter reduction were found in the left circumflex artery (LCX) and in the right coronary artery (RCA). James's coronary heart disease had invaded all the major blood vessels supplying his heart. When physicians are considering treatment options, they need, whenever possible, to have accurate information about the extent and nature of the obstructions. When James's doctor reviewed the angiographic pictures with him, James could clearly see the narrowings and understood that they appeared to jeopardize most of the blood supply to his heart.

In interpreting angiographic images, doctors use the principle that the more myocardium that is potentially jeopardized by obstructed coronary arteries, the worse the prognosis. While we often think of the heart as being supplied by three separate and large coronary arteries (the LAD, LCX, and RCA), the LAD and LCX are actually large branches of a single short left main coronary artery (see plate 1). Narrowing involving the left main coronary artery carries the worst prognosis, because this type of narrowing limits the blood supply to most of the left ventricle and may cause a significant reduction in the pumping capacity of the heart. A complete occlusion of the left main coronary artery is incompatible with life. Narrowing involving this vessel is taken very seriously, because 30 percent of people with a significant narrowing of the left main coronary artery who go without treatment die within eighteen months after diagnosis, and 50 percent die within twenty-four months.

The number of diseased vessels affects the prognosis for each individual. The greater the number of coronary arteries that are affected with significant atherosclerosis, the greater the amount of myocardium that is potentially jeopardized. The more myocardium that is jeopardized, the worse the prognosis is. In general, significant obstruction (more than 70 percent diameter reduction) of only one major coronary artery carries a very good prognosis. The annual mortality rate for patients with this degree of atherosclerosis is 1 to 2 percent per year. Narrowings of the RCA or LCX carry a somewhat better prognosis than if the stenosis is located in the LAD. This difference in mortality is a reflection of the larger amount of myocardium generally supplied by the LAD and the importance of this vessel in maintaining the integrity of the cardiac electrical system.

The location of the narrowing of the LAD makes a big difference. Narrowings that are located near the origin of the artery (and therefore supply a large portion of the left ventricle) carry a worse prognosis than narrowings that are located farther downstream. This difference sets the stage for treating atherosclerotic disease differently when it involves the LAD than when it involves other vessels in the heart. Depending on *which* vessel and the *number* of vessels that are narrowed, your physician can begin to weigh the therapeutic options and decide which one is best for you.

These insights about the significance of the number of diseased coronary arteries were provided by the Coronary Artery Surgery Study (CASS). CASS was conducted in the mid 1980s to assess the relative efficacy of medical therapy versus surgery in patients with obstructive atherosclerotic coronary artery disease. While different types of medical therapies are employed today, the prognostic trends with respect to the extent of coronary heart disease and long-term survival are still valid. In CASS, the four-year survival rate with medical treatment was 92 percent for single-vessel disease, 84 percent for double-vessel disease, and 68 percent for triple-vessel disease. The prognosis, understandably, was worse for patients who already had damage to the heart. These observations underscore the importance, when making therapeutic decisions, of weighing the amount of myocardium at risk. This process is commonly referred to as *assessing the ischemic burden.* In the rest of this chapter and in the next chapter, we examine approaches to reducing the ischemic burden by improving the blood supply.

Balloon Angioplasty

Surgical intervention is the time-honored way to improve a reduced coronary blood supply. In chapter 8 we will see how it is possible to provide the heart with a new blood supply using veins from the leg or elsewhere in the body to form an alternative channel that allows blood to bypass the coronary narrowings (hence the term *coronary artery bypass procedure*). This alternative blood supply is frequently referred to as a *revascularization*. The impact of myocardial revascularization is usually dramatic, improving both the quantity and quality of life for millions of patients around the world.

For years, coronary revascularization was achieved through coronary bypass surgery, appropriately reserved for only the most symptomatic patients or for those at high risk of death. This situation changed in 1977 when Dr. Andreas Gruentzig first reported that certain coronary artery narrowings could be relieved by the expansion of a tiny balloon inside the blood vessel. Today, over one million of these balloon procedures are performed each year in the United States alone. They outnumber coronary bypass procedures by almost two to one and have dramatically changed how doctors approach the treatment of symptomatic coronary heart disease. When James understood that he needed myocardial revascularization, he expressed his strong preference for a balloon procedure.

The technical term for a balloon revascularization procedure is *percutaneous transluminal coronary angioplasty*. The term *percutaneous* is used because the procedure begins with access through the skin. It is not surgery in the traditional sense, because access to the heart is obtained via a needle inserted in the skin, not through an incision. The words *transluminal coronary* mean that the procedure takes place directly inside the blood vessel. *Angioplasty* means blood vessel repair. In essence, a percutaneous transluminal coronary angioplasty (also known as PTCA, or coronary angioplasty) is a coronary artery repair that takes place inside the blood vessel. As with diagnostic coronary arteriography, in a PTCA, a doctor inserts a catheter into the groin and advances it to the opening of the coronary artery. Coronary angioplasty then involves advancing a small wire (measuring 0.014 inches in diameter, about the thickness of a human hair) through the catheter and threading the wire through the partially narrowed coronary artery (see plate 6).

Technological improvements have increased the success rate of the procedure. Nonetheless, it is not always a complete success. If the narrowing is severe or is located deep within the coronary arterial tree or in a vessel that is tortuous, it may take considerable time and skill to advance the tiny wire past the coronary obstruction. Advancing the wire past the obstruction is only the first hurdle involved in a successful coronary angioplasty procedure. This tiny wire must work like a monorail train track, effectively guiding equipment in and out of the heart. With this guide wire in place, a catheter with a sausage-shaped deflated balloon is then advanced over the wire and passed right through the coronary obstruction. If the vessel's diameter is severely reduced, it can be very difficult, if not impossible, to finesse the deflated balloon catheter through the narrowing. Fortunately, in this day and age, the procedure proves impossible for less than 2 percent of patients. Once the coronary balloon has advanced to the point where it is straddling the coronary stenosis, it is inflated at a high pressure, and the obstruction is relieved. The balloon and guide wire are then withdrawn from the body.

What happens to all the atherosclerotic plaque? Initially, it was thought that the plaque was compressed against the blood vessel wall, much like footprints in the snow. But this doesn't make much sense, because atherosclerotic plaque is made of fibrous tissue that may be densely calcified and not very compressible. Another theory was that PTCA stretched the artery to a larger diameter. While initially attractive, this theory is not very accurate, either. An artery that can be easily stretched, like a rubber band, can also easily spring back to its original narrow configuration. What actually happens is that PTCA stretches the coronary artery and in doing so actually stretches the atherosclerotic plaque to the point where the plaque is fractured. To a large extent the blood vessel is actually torn. Thus, PTCA is an act of controlled arterial trauma. It is very much like forcing your finger through a small buttonhole, making the hole larger. This action enlarges the opening, but the material is definitely damaged and is likely to continue to tear. Recognizing that balloon angioplasty traumatizes the blood vessel helps us understand the strengths and weaknesses of this procedure.

Plate 6 depicts the process of coronary angioplasty with cross-sectional views of the coronary artery before, during, and after the procedure. The atherosclerotic plaque is definitely fractured by the procedure. Notice the deep fissures that the balloon dilation has produced in the arterial wall. These fissures now penetrate the endothelial layer and extend into the media layer, where muscular tissue resides. While the blood vessel inner diameter may be larger, it is certainly not perfect. Blood has entered the arterial wall and has seeped beneath the endothelial lining. The act of coronary angioplasty has produced a "blood blister" at the site of the atherosclerotic plaque. In response to the blood pressure within the vessel, the fissures in the blood vessel wall could extend this blood blister in many directions, essentially forming false channels that could grow and eventually compromise the true *lumen* (main channel) of the coronary artery. In an attempt to fix atherosclerotic plaque from the inside out, PTCA actually disrupts the coronary artery, leading to vascular damage, arterial inflammation, and possible thrombus formation. Although the PTCA procedure is initially successful, the damaged coronary artery may clot, causing an acute myocardial infarction—a heart attack. Intracoronary thrombus formation is one of the most serious complications of PTCA.

In its early days, PTCA was neither delicate nor very successful. The technical challenges of advancing a balloon to the obstruction, safely fracturing the atherosclerotic plaque, and then permitting healing without regrowth were formidable. As recently as the early 1990s, coronary balloon angioplasty was associated with a primary success rate of only about 80 percent. There was a very high abrupt thrombosis rate, and emergency coronary bypass surgery was needed for an abrupt thrombosis or an unstable coronary tear in up to 10 percent of all people who had the procedure. Even with initial success, the results of PTCA were not durable. Almost 40 percent of patients had a return of symptoms within six months of their procedure. These disappointing results are certainly not typical of today's procedure. PTCA has undergone considerable evolution over the last ten years (although one does wonder how it survived).

Technical innovations have improved the equipment so that a primary success rate of close to 98 percent is now common. The use of dual platelet inhibition, with both aspirin and clopidogrel, has reduced the chance of abrupt thrombosis to less than 1 percent. Dealing with the return of the coronary obstruction has been a more formidable challenge. Following successful angioplasty, the damaged artery has to heal. In most instances, the artery heals with an internal diameter larger than it had before the PTCA. Unfortunately, in some instances, this healing phase produces intracoronary scar tissue that forms a narrowing that is every bit as severe as the original narrowing. This scar tissue formation is referred to as *restenosis*. For years, coronary restenosis was the Achilles heel of PTCA. Over the years, physicians have used other techniques to combat this process. Attempts to cut out the atherosclerotic plaque (*directional atherectomy*), grind out the plaque (*rotational atherectomy*), burn out the plaque (*laser-assisted angioplasty*), or melt the plaque with radiation (*coronary brachytherapy*) have been disappointing and limited by relatively high complication rates and persistent high restenosis rates. These technologies are still available, but their application to patients with coronary heart disease is limited and is not considered for mainstream use.

The Arrival of Coronary Stents

Coronary balloon angioplasty was forever changed in 1986 with the introduction of intracoronary stents. Intracoronary stents are mesh-like tubes that look similar to the Chinese finger locks that children play with. Compressed over a deflated angioplasty balloon, the stent is advanced over a guide wire to the site of narrowing (plate 7). Made of stainless steel, these flexible tubes are inserted in the coronary artery and expanded at the site of balloon angioplasty. Once in place, they serve as a sort of rigid scaffolding that allows complete expansion of the artery and minimizes any tendency for the traumatized tissue to extend into the vessel and obstruct the flow of blood. By reenforcing the arterial wall, coronary stents virtually eliminated the intra-arterial fissures and false channels that are depicted in plate 6. With this adjunct to PTCA, the risk of abrupt closure of the coronary artery and the need for emergency coronary bypass surgery plummeted. By permitting maximal initial expansion of the artery, coronary stents also maximized myocardial blood flow, resulting in improved clinical outcomes. Assisted by coronary stents, catheter-based procedures soon began to challenge coronary artery bypass grafting as a means of revascularization. A revolution was about to take place within the field of cardiology.

Combining coronary stents with PTCA resulted in a very high initial procedural success rate and excellent clinical results. Unfortunately, despite the use of coronary stents, restenosis continued to plague coronary artery intervention procedures. The reason was that the traumatized coronary artery still needed to heal. The healing process at times produced so much scar tissue that some of it protruded through the stent mesh and narrowed the blood vessel. Coronary angioplasty with metal stent deployment was still associated with an incidence of restenosis of roughly 15 to 20 percent. While significantly lower than the 40 to 50 percent restenosis rate associated with PTCA, it was not yet low enough to challenge coronary artery bypass graft surgery as the preferred means of achieving myocardial revascularization. While coronary restenosis still presented a challenge, the treatment of coronary artery disease was evolving. The availability of coronary stents has made the term PTCA rather obsolete. Stents are now employed in over 80 percent of all coronary intervention procedures. This procedure is sometimes combined with another form of coronary intervention that grinds, cuts, burns or irradiates the atherosclerotic plaque. The generally accepted term for these hybrid procedures is *percutaneous catheter intervention* (PCI). This broader term acknowledges that other treatments may be applied to the heart with a catheter.

The use of coronary stents has reduced the incidence of restenosis in people undergoing PCI. Nonetheless, restenosis continues to occur. Many people are discouraged when they are informed that their PCI has resulted in a restenosis. They may feel that they did something to cause it, but they most certainly did not. The restenotic process is scar tissue that forms within the coronary artery in response to the trauma produced by the coronary intervention procedure itself. It is not caused by the patient's lifestyle or medical noncompliance. Restenosis represents an excessive proliferation of muscle cells and collagen tissue inside the coronary artery. It does not represent an accelerated formation of atherosclerotic plaque. There is a crucial difference between a restenotic coronary lesion and an atherosclerotic plaque.

Unlike atherosclerosis, restenosis following a coronary intervention does not respond to the usual measures of cholesterol reduction, platelet suppression, and inhibition of the vascular inflammation. Preventing the restenotic process could only be accomplished by identifying a biological treatment to impair the growth of scar tissue within the traumatized coronary artery. In retrospect, it is not surprising that cutting, grinding, burning, or irradiating the atherosclerotic plaque was never successful in preventing restenosis. Likewise, virtually every medication that could be ingested, infused, or applied directly to the atherosclerotic plaque has been tried and has failed to impair the restenotic process. For nearly twenty years, restenosis limited the widespread application of PCI. This all changed in the late 1990s.

After years of basic research and some good fortune, two drugs— sirolimus and paclitaxel—were identified as being capable of preventing the excessive tissue growth that characterizes the restenotic process. Sirolimus was initially isolated from a bacterium found in the soil of Easter Island, off the coast of Chile, and paclitaxel was originally purified from the bark of yew trees found in the Brazilian rain forest. Though slightly different in their mechanism of action, both drugs work by entering the nucleus of cells and interfering with the chemical processes responsible for cell replication and growth. By turning off the cells that formed scar tissue in the coronary artery wall, the restenosis process was stopped in its tracks. The Achilles heel of interventional cardiology was all but abolished. The beneficial impact of this development on the field of interventional cardiology has been enormous.

Sirolimus and paclitaxel are both very effective in preventing the cellular proliferation that causes restenosis. Unfortunately, finding the right drug to inhibit scar formation was only one of part of the answer to conquering the problem of restenosis. These medications needed to be administered directly at the site of a coronary stenosis and in doses small enough not to impair cell growth elsewhere in the body. Additional technical innovations devised ways to impregnate stainless steel stents with these medications, deliver these drug-laden stents to the site of coronary angioplasty, and cause the drugs to emerge from the stents and essentially bathe the atherosclerotic plaque in a prolonged and predictable fashion. Today's drug-eluting stents (DES) are technical marvels. Stents are no longer static plugs that hold the coronary artery open. Rather, they are active drug-delivery systems that reside within the heart.

In the field of PCI, drug-eluting stents are only the beginning. Coronary stent technology is rapidly evolving, and soon we may be hearing about biodegradable stents that deliver their drugs and then disappear, or biologically active stents that seed the damaged coronary artery with new (and possibly improved) endothelial cells. Sirolimus and paclitaxel are the two currently available drugs for delivery with a coronary stent. Sirolimus-eluting coronary stents are available as Cypher coronary stents. Paclitaxel-eluting coronary stents are available as Taxus coronary stents.

The reported rates for restenosis using these stents are between 3 and 9 percent, contrasted with the 40 to 50 percent restenosis rates associated with plain PTCA or the 15 to 30 percent restenosis rates associated with bare metal coronary stents. Today's PCI is a far cry from the original procedure developed by Andreas Gruentzig. In just twenty-five years, the catheter-based treatment of atherosclerotic coronary artery disease has evolved to a technique that has a primary success rate near 98 percent, a postprocedural risk of heart attack between 1 and 3 percent, and an acute mortality risk of less than 1 percent. (*Postprocedural,* or *postoperative,* refers to events that occur after the procedure. In general, the postprocedural risk period is twelve to twenty-four hours postprocedure. *Periprocedural,* or *perioperative,* means before and after the procedure takes place.) It is no wonder that James, like many patients, inquired about a catheter-based procedure as a mean of treating his coronary heart disease. The widespread availability of PCI has revolutionized the treatment of coronary heart disease, but as good as PCI currently is, it remains an imperfect procedure that is still associated with some significant risks. It is not appropriate for everyone.

An intracoronary stent is a foreign body that remains permanently implanted within the coronary artery wall. Your body does not reject this foreign material in the way that it would reject a transplanted organ. Rather, the stent is incorporated into the blood vessel wall much like a splinter can be lodged under your skin. With time, the stent becomes biologically inert, effectively invisible to the watchful eyes of the immune and coagulation systems. For it to become inert, the metal struts of the stent must become covered with the protective endothelial lining. Until the endothelial lining of the coronary artery is reformed around the stent, there remains a tendency for blood clots to form on the stent, which would cause a heart attack. The tendency to form blood clots soon after coronary stent insertion is referred to as *subacute thrombosis*. Subacute thrombosis can occur suddenly, without prior symptoms, and has been associated with a mortality rate of 15 to 40 percent. Subacute thrombosis is a serious problem and may represent the new Achilles heel of coronary stent use.

With bare metal stents, the incidence of subacute thrombosis is approximately 1 percent, although this risk is increased with the number of stents deployed and as the stent size decreases. Subacute thrombosis occurs because the metal struts of the stent activate circulating platelets. Therefore the risk of subacute thrombosis can be significantly reduced if the patient takes both aspirin and clopidogrel to aggressively inhibit platelets. For bare metal stents, platelet inhibition treatment generally lasts 1 to 3 months. During this period, the vascular endothelium grows like ivy on a wall, eventually completely covering the intracoronary stent. With the stent fully endothelialized, the chance of having a subacute thrombosis of the stent is almost nil and the antiplatelet therapy can safely be discontinued.

Drug-eluting stents are entirely different from bare metal stents. Recent clinical data have suggested that DES may be associated with a higher and significantly longer period of risk for subacute thrombosis. While the data are not entirely clear, the risk of stent thrombosis may extend to periods longer than a year. We are not certain why this is true, but because the mechanism action for the drugs used in DES is to inhibit cell growth and replication, it makes sense that these drugs, in addition to inhibiting the growth of smooth muscle cells (the principle component of a restenotic scar), may also inhibit the growth of protective endothelial cells. Several studies using *coronary angioscopy* (a fiberoptic telescope that can be inserted directly into the coronary arteries) have confirmed that incomplete endothelialization of DES is indeed associated with subacute thrombosis. Fortunately, the prolonged use of aspirin and clopidogrel seems to reduce this risk significantly. If you have had a DES inserted, you should not stop taking aspirin or clopidogrel without the advice and consent of your physician.

When Is a Stent Appropriate Treatment?

In appropriate patients and in the correct clinical setting, the insertion of a coronary stent is a major advance in the treatment of coronary heart disease. However, not every patient with a narrowed coronary artery requires a percutaneous catheter intervention and a coronary stent. Since they became available in 2004, drug-eluting stents have fueled an explosive growth in the application of PCI to coronary heart disease. This growth has placed a huge financial burden on the health care system without a clear-cut beneficial effect on patient survival.

As we saw in chapter 6, medical therapy for coronary heart disease evolves at a rapid pace. In many instances, drug therapy can be undertaken with a high degree of success and minimal risk to the patient. There is likewise little question that a PCI can relieve symptoms of angina in most patients. But how can we weigh one treatment over another? Clinical trials take years to develop and to enroll patients while both forms of treatment continue to evolve. Direct comparisons between these two forms of therapy are difficult to conduct, because it is impossible to blind investigators to the form of therapy being administered, and considerable selection bias is inevitable.

The Clinical Outcomes Utilizing Revascularization and Aggressive Drug Evaluation (COURAGE) trial was the latest attempt to compare the relative efficacy of conservative medical therapy and PCI. Published in 2007, this study randomized 2,287 patients with angina pectoris treatment with either PCI plus optimal medical therapy or optimal medical therapy alone. Patients were followed for 2.5 to 7 years. At the end of the study, there were no significant differences between the treatment groups with respect to death, nonfatal heart attack, or stroke. Patients treated with PCI initially had fewer symptoms of angina, but this difference was no longer apparent after five years of follow-up. Nearly one-third of all patients initially randomized to receive medical therapy required either PCI or coronary bypass surgery for worsening symptoms. Nonetheless, this study received great attention in the lay press as a possible rebuke of the benefits of PCI for the treatment of coronary heart disease.

The results of the COURAGE trial are not surprising, because placing a metal stent over one small part of the coronary artery cannot possibly provide long-term protection against additional atherosclerotic plaque formation or subsequent plaque rupture at another location within the heart. Atherosclerosis is a systemic process characterized by the infiltration of lipid-laden macrophages, inflammation, and thrombus formations—and PCI gets rid of the symptoms but does not treat the disease. The successful treatment of atherosclerosis is a long-term treatment that requires much more than a band-aid over the plaque.

The COURAGE trial is not alone in highlighting the limitations of treatment with PCI. While many clinical trials have documented the efficacy of PCI in relieving the symptoms of angina, no clinical trial has shown that PCI has a beneficial impact on long-term survival in patients. Some caution should be exhibited before extrapolating the results of COURAGE and similar trials to all patients with coronary heart disease.

Most of the clinical trials comparing medical therapy with PCI enroll mildly symptomatic patients who are otherwise healthy and have atherosclerosis limited to either single-vessel coronary artery disease or double-vessel coronary artery disease and who have well-preserved cardiac function. In the COURAGE trial, only 5 percent of the eligible patients were actually enrolled; this is because physicians and patients alike are often reluctant to be randomized to receive a specific form of treatment when they are "sure" of the relative merits of one or the other treatment arms. Obtaining clinical information that is relevant to the diversity of clinical situations that are routinely faced is very difficult. Each patient and his or her clinical situation must be considered in the context of overall health. There may be underlying medical conditions that raise the risk of PCI and make it an inferior alternative to medical therapy (medications), and there may be conditions that make medical therapy inferior to a revascularization procedure. Your physician will help guide you through the decision-making process and will take many factors into account.

Because of the size of some arteries or of the cardiac structures they supply, some arteries may have a disproportionate impact on prognosis. As noted earlier, this is true of the left anterior descending coronary artery. Some studies suggest that significant atherosclerotic disease of this particular vessel may be better managed with some form of revascularization procedure. The significance of the LAD probably is related to its size. It is often the largest of all the coronary arteries and arguably the most important one because it supplies the portion of the heart that houses many of the electrical circuits that control cardiac contraction. For most other arteries, PCI should be reserved for the control of anginal symptoms that do not respond to conventional therapy or for patients in an unfavorable prognostic category after noninvasive cardiac testing. The debate over whether medications or revascularization are superior as the initial treatment of coronary heart disease has been going on for quite some time and will likely continue as new methods for achieving myocardial revascularization emerge. An equally lively debate centers on the relative merits of bypass surgery and catheter intervention as the preferred means of performing coronary revascularization.

All Revascularization Procedures Are Not Created Equally

In some circumstances, medical therapy is decidedly unsatisfactory, and the person needs a new or improved blood supply. This is certainly true in patients with a stenosis of the left main coronary artery; patients with multivessel coronary artery disease; patients who have compromised left ventricular function; and patients with diabetes. For people in each of these populations, a myocardial revascularization has been shown to be superior to standard medical therapy. Traditionally, the myocardial revascularization procedure has been coronary artery bypass graft (CABG) surgery, and a wealth of clinical data support the use of surgical revascularization in these patient groups.

With the success and widespread availability of drug-eluting coronary stents, it may seem reasonable to extend these data to percutaneous catheter interventions, but doing so may not be advisable.

Coronary stenting, like coronary bypass surgery, has its own set of risks and benefits. For every intracoronary stent that is inserted, there is a risk of additional arterial damage, blood clot formation, and restenosis. As the number of stents inserted increases, the risk for these events accumulates. With the insertion of multiple stents, the risk of PCI may increase so that there is no advantage compared with coronary bypass surgery in a specific patient. Likewise, the insertion of coronary stents requires the administration of potent anticoagulants and iodine contrast agents. There is a risk of bleeding and renal failure that increases significantly with age and with certain medical conditions like diabetes. Weighing the risks and benefits of these procedures has been an elusive goal as the technology and safety of both PCI and coronary bypass surgery have continued to improve. Most of the clinical trials comparing the efficacy of multivessel PCI versus CABG took place before drug-eluting stents were available. Accordingly, a direct comparison of these procedures is difficult. Keep this distinction in mind as we review some of the clinical data.

There are several large clinical trials comparing the efficacy of multivessel PCI with CABG. All of them are challenged by an attempt to ensure that the two treatment groups have patients with identical clinical characteristics, including age and gender as well as the nature and severity of the atherosclerotic disease, the overall condition of the left ventricle, and the prevalence of other medical conditions such as diabetes and renal failure. As you can imagine, controlling for all these variables can be challenging. The ARTS group trial of about a decade ago is one of the better prospective, randomized clinical trials comparing PCI and CABG in similar patient populations.

The ARTS group trial was designed to examine the clinical outcomes in patients with multivessel coronary artery disease who were prospectively randomized to treatment with either conventional coronary bypass surgery (CABG) or percutaneous catheter intervention (PCI) with a *bare metal* coronary stent. This was a fairly large study, enrolling 1,205 patients, with follow-up of more than five years available for both groups of patients.

The outcome of the ARTS trial was very much as expected. There was no statistically significant difference in mortality at one year (PCI 2.5 percent vs. CABG 2.8 percent), at three years (PCI 3.7 percent vs. CABG 4.6 percent), or at five years (PCI 3.7 percent vs. CABG 4.6 percent). Likewise, there was no difference between the groups for the combined clinical outcome of death, nonfatal heart attack, or stroke at one, three, or five years. The ARTS trial, with several other randomized and nonrandomized clinical trials comparing these two therapies, suggested that when revascularization was clinically indicated, PCI was similar to CABG with respect to the usual clinical endpoints. There were several significant exceptions, however. First was the observation that despite the placement of one or more coronary stents, the derived clinical benefit of PCI was not as durable as that of CABG. Many patients undergoing PCI with an initially uneventful procedure required a second procedure during the five-year period of observation. In ARTS, 30 percent of patients randomized to PCI required a repeat revascularization procedure as compared to only 8.8 percent of those initially treated with CABG. In the PCI-treated group, the additional revascularization procedure was more often than not CABG rather than an attempt at a second PCI. For the patients enrolled in this study, PCI with bare metal stents delayed but did not eliminate the eventual need for surgical revascularization.

The ARTS trial highlighted another shortcoming of multivessel PCI. Not every patient randomized to PCI received a complete revascularization. In some patients who were randomized to PCI, not all significant coronary obstructions were relieved because, either due to complex anatomy or other technical reasons, a coronary stent simply could not be inserted in the designated target vessel. To be fair, this technical limitation is also applicable to CABG, although not as often. In the ARTS trial, 84 percent of patients randomized to CABG received a complete revascularization while 71 percent of patients randomized to PCI received a complete revascularization. After one year, patients who were randomized to PCI and were incompletely revascularized often required a second revascularization procedure. Again, this was usually bypass surgery. The ARTS trial also confirmed the observations of other trials that people with diabetes respond poorly to PCI. For people with diabetes, the one-year event-free survival rate (freedom from death, heart attack, or repeat revascularization) was significantly lower in patients undergoing PCI (63 percent) versus CABG (84 percent). This difference was principally driven by a much higher need for repeat revascularization in the PCI group. While coronary stents are a major innovation in the treatment of coronary heart disease, the ARTS trial underscored the importance of complete revascularization and the vulnerability of people with diabetes to the restenotic process.

The initial ARTS trial was conducted in the era before drug-eluting stents, and it will take several years to conduct similar randomized prospective trials with the relatively new DES. Some insight into the potential effects of DES may be gleaned from an analysis of the ARTS II registry. In this nonrandomized study, patients received DES for various indications and were prospectively enrolled in a database. This DES-treated group was then retrospectively (looking back) compared to the CABG-treated group assembled in the original ARTS trial. This comparison was made between groups of patients treated at very different points in time. There are many potential risks and biases introduced with this kind of study. Nonetheless, some useful observations can be made.

The recent ARTS II registry data suggest that PCI with drug-eluting stents has made considerable progress in the treatment of multivessel coronary heart disease. Once again, there was no statistically significant difference with respect to mortality between the PCI- and CABG-treated groups. You will recall that in the ARTS trial, the greatest limitation of bare metal stent use was the eventual need for a repeat revascularization procedure. The use of drug-eluting stents closed the gap in the need for revascularization. In ARTS II, only 8.5 percent of PCI treated patients required a second revascularization procedure within the first year (vs. 21.3 percent in ARTS).

The ARTS II registry data suggest that drug-eluting stents offer promise as a treatment for multivessel coronary artery disease, although for some patient subgroups, revascularization with PCI may be inferior to conventional CABG. This includes patients with diabetes and patients with significant narrowing of the left main coronary artery. For other patients with multivessel coronary artery disease, CABG may be clinically equivalent to PCI with respect to outcome, the latter offering a distinct advantage with respect to patient comfort and convenience.

The long-term consequences of DES are not yet known. Additional studies are needed. The Synergy between PCI with Taxus and Cardiac Surgery (SYNTAX) trial is currently under way and should be completed by 2012. This and several other similar studies will shed light on this topic. For the time being, myocardial revascularization with PCI cannot be viewed as an equivalent to conventional CABG for patients with obstructions of the left main coronary artery or significant obstructions of three or more coronary arteries. This may be particularly true for patients with diabetes or patients in whom a complete revascularization cannot be obtained.

Drug-eluting stents have helped and will continue to help millions of patients. Their principal benefit is that they minimize the chance of coronary restenosis. The current guidelines for DES indicate that they should be reserved for use in patients where the risk of restenosis is high, including all people with diabetes, all patients with long, complex coronary stenoses, and patients whose atherosclerotic lesions involve a *bifurcation* of vessels or small diameter coronary arteries. A bifurcation is the situation where a blood vessel branches in a Y configuration. This represents a challenge in PCI because successful coverage with stents may require three separate stents or the positioning of one stent across the opening of the other (called a *stent jail*). The presence of a coronary lesion that involves a bifurcation represents a technical challenge and a higher risk of restenosis or subacute thrombosis.

The use of DES in people with narrowed coronary bypass grafts or in someone with an acute myocardial infarction is controversial. Coronary bypass grafts do not develop typical atherosclerosis, and therefore the antiproliferative effects of the eluted drugs may not be as striking. Given the increased risk of subacute thrombosis, there is some concern about placing DES in an acutely thrombosed coronary artery. Several clinical research trials are under way to address these issues.

While the use of DES in some situations is open to debate, there is little question that PCI is a very effective way to treat a heart attack. A heart attack occurs when an atherosclerotic plaque ulcerates and an occlusive thrombus forms at the site of endothelial injury. Deprived of oxygen-rich blood, the myocardium soon begins to suffocate and eventually become irreversibly injured.

Treating a Person Who Is Having a Heart Attack

With the occlusion of the coronary artery, the life of myocardial tissue is endangered and will die unless it is rescued. As time passes, the lack of nutrients will cause tissue death. Irreversible damage to cardiac muscle begins after roughly forty minutes of coronary occlusion. After six hours of coronary occlusion, most if not all the muscle supplied by this artery is irreversibly damaged. This six-hour time frame represents a window of opportunity to treat a heart attack through *reperfusion therapy*. Reperfusion therapy means the restoration of blood flow to the obstructed coronary artery. The restoration of coronary blood flow will minimize the amount of myocardial damage. The earlier the restoration, the less the accumulated myocardial damage. Less myocardial damage translates into fewer patient deaths and less disability. Reperfusion therapy limits myocardial damage, unquestionably improving patient outcomes.

The value of reperfusion therapy was brought to light in an Italian study called GISSI, in which patients having a heart attack were randomized to receive either conventional medical management (of aspirin, heparin, nitrates, and beta-blocking drugs) or *thrombolytic therapy* (*thrombus*, clot, + *lysis*, dissolve, often referred to as clot-busting). All the drugs that dissolve clots are called *thrombolytic agents*. Sometimes the more precise term *fibrinolytic agents* is used, because these drugs dissolve clots by dissolving the fibrin strands that hold clots together. Thrombolytic agents, fibrinolytic agents, and *plasminogen activators* all refer to the same group of drugs that dissolve clots. In the GISSI study, the blood clot–dissolving agent streptokinase was used. The results of this landmark study are depicted in figure 7.1.

What does figure 7.1 show? First, that patients who received thrombolytic therapy had a lower mortality rate than those who received standard (and very good) medical therapy. Opening an acutely occluded coronary artery resulted in a significant reduction in mortality. Second, the figure shows that the earlier the coronary artery is

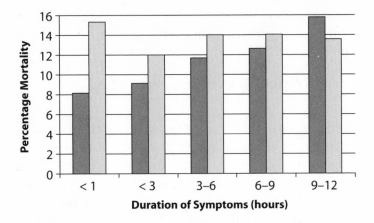

FIGURE 7.1. The impact of thrombolytic therapy. Dark bars represent patients treated with intravenous streptokinase (thrombolytic therapy); light bars represent patients treated with standard medical therapy. This figure demonstrates the beneficial impact of thrombolytic therapy for patients having a heart attack. Note the significant improvement in survival associated with thrombolytic therapy. Also note the impact of *early* treatment on outcome. The benefit of treatment is effectively lost if it is administered after six to nine hours of symptoms. (Adapted from "GISSI Trial," *Lancet* 1 (1986): 397–402.)

opened after the onset of symptoms of a heart attack, the greater the reduction in mortality. Treatment within the first hour of symptoms cut mortality in half. Six hours after the onset of symptoms, there was no appreciable reduction in mortality provided by thrombolytic therapy.

The GISSI trial took place over twenty years ago and was considered groundbreaking. Today reperfusion of an acutely occluded coronary artery has become standard therapy for the treatment of heart attack. The methods used to achieve successful reperfusion have evolved considerably. Streptokinase (which was used in GISSI) has been replaced by any one of several more potent clot-busting drugs that can open an occluded coronary artery close to 80 percent of the time. The intravenous administration of *tissue plasminogen activators*, as they are now called, is only one means of reperfusing an acutely occluded coronary artery. It is now also possible to mechanically recanalize the blood vessel with a coronary balloon angioplasty and the insertion of a coronary stent. Identifying the most advantageous method of reperfusion is one of the great debates of cardiovascular medicine.

The debate goes something like this. A percutanous coronary intervention may open an occluded coronary artery close to 98 percent of the time. Thrombolytic therapy is successful in doing so only 80 percent of the time. Not only is PCI more likely to open an occluded artery, it tends to provide a more effective means of reperfusion. The blood flow following a PCI is often graded to be more brisk than after thrombolytic therapy. There are numerous clinical trials comparing the relative efficacy of thrombolytic therapy and PCI. All have demonstrated the superiority of PCI with respect to the quantity and quality of restored myocardial blood flow.

In addition to being a more effective reperfusion strategy, PCI seems to be a safer procedure. Thrombolytic therapy, while very successful in dissolving coronary thrombus, is also very successful in dissolving thrombus that may be located elsewhere in the body. As a result, thrombolytic therapy is associated with a significant risk of bleeding. The most feared location for bleeding is within the brain, often referred to as an *intracranial hemorrhage* or a *hemorrhagic stroke*. The use of thrombolytic drugs is generally associated with a risk of intracranial bleeding of close to 1 percent. This risk may be substantially increased in elderly people, people with a prior history of a stroke, people with a history of hypertension, and people with a small body mass (predominantly women).

In addition to the risk of intracranial bleeding, the use of thrombolytic agents carries a risk of nonfatal bleeding elsewhere. A partially healed peptic ulcer can easily rebleed. What was a small bruise can suddenly turn into a very large one. The risk of significant nonfatal bleeding may approach 5 percent of all patients treated with thrombolytic therapy. The risk of intracranial bleeding associated with PCI is near 0 percent and the risk of nonfatal bleeding somewhat less than 5 percent. Thus it would seem that PCI is a more effective and safer method of achieving myocardial reperfusion. So what is there to debate? Shouldn't everyone who enters the emergency room with an acute myocardial infarction be treated with an emergency PCI as the preferred method of reperfusion? Not so fast.

PCI is not universally available. It requires access to a cardiac catheterization facility and the availability of skilled operators. Such resources are available in less than 20 percent of hospitals in the United

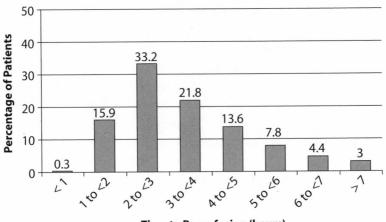

Time to Reperfusion (hours)

FIGURE 7.2. Time to treatment in patients with a heart attack treated with PCI. This figure depicts data from several thousand patients who came to hospitals for treatment of an acute myocardial infarction. Most patients come for treatment after experiencing symptoms for two to three hours. In fact, only 16 percent of patients seek medical care after having symptoms for only two hours or less. Given the link between early treatment and survival, we can see that most people wait too long before seeking medical attention, depriving themselves of effective treatment. (Redrawn from original in B. K. Nallamothu et al., "Times to Treatment in Transfer Patients Undergoing Primary Percutaneous Coronary Intervention in the United States: National Registry of Myocardial Infarction (NRMI)—3/4 analysis," *Circulation* 111 (2005): 761–67.)

States. Performing a PCI on a person who is having a heart attack is very difficult and cannot be done by anyone or everywhere. People who come to a hospital that does not have a cardiac catheterization facility are often transferred to other facilities for their emergency PCI. This invariably introduces a delay in achieving successful reperfusion. In studies where thrombolytic therapy was directly compared with mechanical reperfusion via PCI, this delay in treatment was close to one hour. In the treatment of a heart attack, the loss of time means loss of muscle. As a result, despite more effective reperfusion, the mortality benefit of PCI-mediated reperfusion is modest (when compared with thrombolytics). Most studies show that patients treated with PCI, despite having a clearly higher rate of reperfusion, have only 1 percent lower mortality than those treated with thrombolytic therapy. The importance of early treatment of an acute myocardial infarction with any form of reperfusion therapy cannot be overemphasized. Unfortunately, current data suggest that most patients experience a considerable delay in receiving this life-saving treatment.

Figure 7.2 depicts the time to apply mechanical reperfusion to 4,278 patients having an acute myocardial infarction who arrived at 419 different hospitals across the United States. A minority of patients received successful reperfusion within two hours of the onset of symptoms. Compare this time-to-treatment data with the time-to-treatment and mortality data depicted in figure 7.1. An alarmingly high number of patients receive reperfusion therapy after the window of therapeutic opportunity has closed. Much of the delay depicted in figure 7.2 occurred because of the time it took to transfer the patient to a hospital with cardiac catheterization capabilities. To significantly change mortality associated with acute myocardial infarction will require expediting the application of reperfusion therapy. The current guidelines for treatment of an acute myocardial infarction are to achieve a "door to balloon time" of ninety minutes or less. If this cannot be achieved, the administration of intravenous thrombolytic therapy is recommended.

A heart attack can be successfully treated with either thrombolytic therapy or mechanical reperfusion with PCI. What is important is to obtain life-saving treatment in a timely manner. Don't deny or ignore your symptoms. If you have new or unusual symptoms that might be suggestive of a heart attack, seek attention immediately at the nearest hospital. The physicians there will determine whether your symptoms are related to your heart and whether thrombolytic therapy or mechanical reperfusion with PCI is best for you.

In answering James's original questions, we can say that the appropriateness of a balloon procedure, or PCI, depends on many factors, including the patient's coronary anatomy and general health, and the physician's experience. PCI was not an option for James, who had severe multivessel coronary artery disease that is best treated with coronary bypass surgery. The cumulative risk of performing PCI in all of the complex stenoses in James's heart increased his risk for complication to the point where PCI was comparable to coronary bypass surgery. Nonetheless, James and his family were understandably concerned. Open-heart surgery is frightening and is more complicated than PCI. However, the short-term and long-term results of coronary bypass surgery in most patients are excellent. In the next chapter, we find out what's involved in this surgery.

EIGHT

When Is Surgery the Best Treatment?

James needed a coronary bypass operation, and he knew that he was facing a major surgical procedure. Understandably, James and his family had concerns about the prospect of what many people call "open-heart surgery." Nobody wants to have surgery, especially one in which surgeons need to open your heart. And heart surgery does carry risks. But many people have misconceptions about the technical aspects, clinical benefits, and risks of cardiac surgery. James and his doctor talked about coronary bypass surgery at some length, discussing the benefits of the procedure and dispelling many of his misconceptions. In the right patients, with the right reasons for surgery (what doctors call *clinical indications*), coronary bypass surgery can truly be life saving. Anyone living with coronary heart disease ought to understand the strengths and weaknesses of all the options for treating the disease. Coronary bypass surgery is an incredibly important therapeutic option—sometimes it is the only option that offers the hope of saving a life.

James's cardiac catheterization confirmed that his heart was being supplied by coronary arteries that were severely narrowed by atherosclerotic plaque in multiple locations. James's disease could not be safely and effectively treated with a coronary balloon angioplasty with stenting (discussed in chapter 7) because there were too many narrowings, located in anatomically difficult locations. Collectively, these narrowings limited the blood supply to a significant portion of James's left ventricle, and the ischemic burden caused by his narrowed coronary arteries placed him in an unfavorable prognostic category for treatment with medications alone. Without a better blood supply to his heart, James would continue to have symptoms of angina, but the crucial issue was that he would be at significant risk for a future heart attack and death. He clearly needed a better blood supply to the heart, and the only way to provide one was to intervene surgically.

What Happens in Surgery?

A coronary bypass operation does exactly what it claims: the existing coronary blockages are left in place and new blood vessels are surgically installed to establish an alternative route for blood to use in traveling to the heart. These new blood vessels serve as effective detours that bypass the existing obstructions. In many ways, these bypass vessels function like the collateral blood vessels described in chapter 5, except that they are larger and thus more effective in delivering blood to the heart. Thinking of collateral blood vessels as dirt road detours, bypass vessels are the equivalent of super highways.

Creating alternative pathways for blood, while simple in concept, is difficult to achieve in practice. Putting new pathways in place requires stopping the heart for a period. Years ago, this led to technical innovations and new machines to take over the function of the heart and lungs while the heart was stopped. New drugs also had to be devised to protect and support the body's functioning during and after surgery. In addition, a select group of surgeons and other physicians worked to develop the skills to intervene microscopically in the body's most vital organ with life temporarily suspended.

Forty years of technical innovations and a generation of cardiac surgeons have transformed this procedure to the point where it is now a relatively safe therapeutic option for many people with coronary heart disease. However, even though coronary bypass surgery has become fairly commonplace, it is still a major surgical procedure. Coronary bypass surgery requires a team of highly trained and specialized physicians, nurses, and technicians working together to ensure the patient's safety and a speedy recovery. Before examining the details of the surgery and variations of the surgery, let's consider an overview of what takes place in the operating room and beyond.

Like all types of cardiac surgery, coronary bypass surgery requires general anesthesia. This means that you are soundly and deeply asleep for the entire procedure. It is the *cardiac anesthesiologist*'s job to keep you in a deep sleep state and to monitor your body's systems during surgery. The cardiac anesthesiologist is a physician specially trained to provide anesthesia during this kind of surgery.

While under general anesthesia, all patients require some help breathing. Breathing is assisted with a machine called a *mechanical ventilator,* or *respirator.* Several times each minute, this machine injects oxygen-rich air into the lungs, ensuring that the body has all the oxygen it needs during surgery. To connect the patient to the respirator, the anesthesiologist places a small tube, called an *endotracheal tube,* through the mouth and down the throat. This tube, which is connected to the respirator, is a source of concern for many patients. Nearly always, the endotracheal tube stays in place for only a few hours after surgery is completed. It is removed once the patient is awake enough or strong enough to breathe on his or her own. In fact, many patients who have had coronary bypass surgery never remember having an endotracheal tube in place.

Everyone undergoing major surgery will need an endotracheal tube for at least a short period. Some patients, because of the health of their lungs, may need the tube in place a bit longer. The tube makes sure that the patient has enough oxygen and that the airway is protected against oral secretions inadvertently going down the "wrong pipe." While prolonged use of an endotracheal tube has definite benefits, it also poses some risks. These include irritation to the vocal cords or soft tissues of the mouth and throat. For these reasons, there is a limit to how long the endotracheal tube can be left in place. For patients who may require the use of a respirator for an extended period, a *tracheostomy* may be performed. When the patient needs help getting enough oxygen or avoiding aspirating secretions, the tracheostomy has several advantages over an endotracheal tube.

A tracheostomy is a small hole made by a surgeon in the trachea through the lower portion of the neck. Because it uses a much smaller tube for ventilation and bypasses the vocal cords and the soft tissues in the mouth, a tracheostomy tube is much safer and more comfortable for the patient than an endotracheal tube. If needed, it can be left in place for a longer time, allowing the patient to recover. A tracheostomy is an uncommonly used but valuable tool to assist some patients in their recovery following surgery. When the tracheostomy is no longer needed, the tube is removed, allowing the small hole to heal. The overwhelming majority of patients who undergo coronary bypass surgery will not require a tracheostomy.

To perform traditional coronary bypass surgery, the surgeon must have full access to the heart and great vessels inside the chest. Access is obtained by making a surgical incision over the *sternum* (the breastbone). The sternum is then divided, and the heart is exposed. To attach the bypass grafts to the heart, the heart is usually stopped (*cardioplegia*) and a cardiopulmonary bypass (CPB) machine (an incredible machine often called the *heart-lung machine*) takes over the job of the heart and lungs. During this period, the cardiac anesthesiologist and cardiac surgeon monitor all the body's functions very closely. During CPB, blood is diverted out of the body to the heart-lung machine, where it is cooled, resupplied with oxygen, and then pumped through the body at an appropriate blood pressure. Because the body is cooled, a state of suspended animation is created, during which the body's metabolic requirements are markedly reduced. While the heart is stopped during CPB, the heart-lung machine takes over the function of these vital organs, keeping the patient physically stable throughout the procedure.

With the heart still, the surgeon is able to carefully sew new blood vessels along the blocked coronary arteries, creating the coronary bypass. Plate 8 depicts a heart with several types of coronary bypass grafts in place. (These grafts are taken from the leg or another location, as discussed later in this chapter.) There is no question that this is difficult surgery. For one thing, the diameter of the coronary arteries is only one to four millimeters. That's roughly the height of one of the capital letters in this text. Using glasses that magnify microscopic views, the surgeon is able to seamlessly sew these tiny blood vessels together with microscopic suture that is about as fine as human hair.

The suturing must be done very skillfully. If the sutures are sewn too loosely, the connection between the blood vessels may leak, leading to bleeding around the heart. If the sutures are too tight, the attachment may narrow, introducing a new obstruction to coronary blood flow. The successful connection of the bypass grafts and the coronary artery is referred to as an anastomosis (ə-nas´-tə-mō´-sis). Establishing a successful anastomosis between the bypass graft and the coronary arteries is one of the most crucial steps in the coronary bypass operation. This delicate tailoring is aided by the heart not moving during this part of the procedure. This temporary period of cardiac arrest, while of great benefit during the creation of the anastomosis, has some drawbacks as well. (An approach to surgery that avoids the period of cardiac arrest is described later in this chapter.)

A few words about terminology are in order here. Everyone has heard of single, double, triple, or even quadruple coronary bypass surgery. These terms refer to the number of new conduits that have been installed. Plate 8 depicts a heart that has undergone a triple coronary bypass procedure. It's easy to understand why someone would think that a double-vessel bypass procedure would be twice as risky as a single-vessel procedure, and that a triple- or quadruple-vessel procedure is riskier yet. This is not necessarily true. Most surgical risk is brought about by the use of general anesthesia, the opening of the chest, and the use of cardiopulmonary bypass. The number of vessels bypassed slightly extends the duration of the procedure but does not significantly increase the risks to the patient.

One of the major drawbacks of traditional coronary bypass surgery is that to divert blood to the cardiopulmonary bypass machine, the cardiac surgeon must manipulate and ultimately clamp and insert tubes into the aorta, the body's largest blood vessel. Another drawback is that to prevent the blood from forming blood clots while it is out of the body, large amounts of anticoagulant medications must be given, increasing the risk of postoperative bleeding. Despite these limitations, the overwhelming majority of coronary bypass procedures performed today use cardioplegia (temporary cessation of cardiac activity) and temporary use of cardiopulmonary bypass.

Once the new coronary bypass grafts are in place, the body is slowly rewarmed. The heart is restarted and once again pumps blood throughout the body. The cardiopulmonary bypass machine is no longer needed, and the tubes diverting blood out of the body are removed. The sternum and the skin are closed, and the patient is transferred to the intensive care unit (ICU).

Patients newly out of surgery are attached to complex devices and are given various medications for support in the early postoperative period, and the ICU is the best setting for closely monitoring devices and medications. In the ICU, patients receive personalized and intensive care by a team of health care professionals who are expert in providing this care. Many patients' families are shocked by all the tubes and machines that are connected to their loved ones. They can rest assured that this is standard procedure in the early recovery period, and that many of these support items will be removed in the first few hours after surgery. Most patients spend one to two days in the ICU. They then spend three to five days convalescing in the cardiac step-down unit.

In the step-down unit, care is focused on improving lung function and eliminating excess body fluid gained during surgery. All open-heart surgery patients have these needs, which do not signal the development of congestive heart failure or pneumonia. Likewise, most patients experience some soreness at the site of sternal incision, but there is generally not much postoperative pain. Nearly everyone who has a sore breastbone tries to avoid taking deep breaths, but avoiding deep breathing is not a good thing for anyone who has had surgery. The nursing staff and respiratory therapist will work very hard to make sure that patients *do* breathe deeply and clear their lungs of any secretions. This is the best way to prevent pneumonia after surgery and to assist in recovery.

While the patient is in the step-down unit, the electrical rhythm of the heart is continuously monitored. As many as 30 percent of all patients develop a rapid heart rate following their coronary bypass procedure. This cardiac rhythm, referred to as *atrial fibrillation,* is more of a nuisance than a danger, although the rapid heart rate and palpitations associated with atrial fibrillation are frightening to some patients. Generally, this rapid heart rate is effectively treated with medications and resolves in a short period. While the emergence of this heart rhythm may prolong the hospitalization a day or two, it should not be considered a setback at all.

After five to seven days in the hospital, most patients are ready to go home. By the time they are discharged from the hospital, they should be able walk and move around on their own. Some patients may require periodic home visits by nurses to examine surgical incisions and assist with administering medications. In the early recovery period, patients may have disturbed sleep and notice changes in dietary habits. A weight loss of five to ten pounds is not uncommon. Many patients experience ups and downs in emotions and may cry easily or be irritable at times, but these mood shifts generally settle down relatively quickly.

Most patients rapidly progress to regular activities while they convalesce at home, generally for three or four weeks. During this time, patients are prohibited from doing any heavy lifting, vigorous exercise, or driving. *These are very important restrictions,* not because the heart is weak but to allow the separated sternum to fully heal. One month after coronary bypass surgery, most patients are ready and able to pursue a full and vigorous life.

Putting Risk in Perspective

Over the past thirty years, technical innovations have dramatically reduced the risks of coronary bypass surgery. This reduction in risk has occurred despite the trend to operate on older and sicker patients. In general, the perioperative mortality rate (death around the time of the procedure) for coronary bypass surgery is between 2 and 5 percent. The risks of coronary bypass surgery depend on several variables. Risk-prediction algorithms are used to assess the risks of coronary bypass surgery, but all these tools are limited by the age of the database and variations in the techniques and surgical experience of the contributing centers. In the United States, algorithms developed by the Society of Thoracic Surgeons are most commonly used. The EuroSCORE is a similar algorithm developed in Europe and may be slightly more predictive of future outcomes (see table 8.1).

These mortality predictions should not be taken literally. They refer to *groups* of patients, in a statistical sense. Each patient is unique and may have an operative risk that is lower or higher than would be predicted by any of the surgical algorithms. Nonetheless, table 8.1 is useful in underscoring the contribution of specific comorbidities to the relative risk of cardiac surgery.

Clearly, age is a significant risk factor in determining perioperative

TABLE 8.1   *European System for Cardiac Operative Risk Evaluation:*
EuroSCORE Risk Index

Predictor	Definition	Risk Points
Age	Points for every 5 years over age 60	1
Sex	Female	1
Chronic pulmonary disease	Long-term use of bronchodilators or steroids for lung disease	1
Extracardiac vascular disease	Any one or more of the following: claudication carotid stenosis > 50% previous or planned intervention on the abdominal aorta, limb arteries, or carotid arteries	2
Neurological dysfunction	Disease severely affecting the ability to ambulate in daily functioning	2
Previous cardiac surgery	Requiring an opening of the pericardium	3
Renal function	Creatinine > 2.3 mg/dl preoperatively	2
Active endocarditis	If under antibiotic treatment at time of surgery	3
Critical preoperative state	Any one or more of the following: ventricular tachycardia, fibrillation, or aborted sudden cardiac death preoperative cardiac massage preoperative mechanical ventilation preoperative inotropic support need for preoperative intra-aortic balloon counterpulsation preoperative acute renal failure	3
Unstable angina	Rest angina requiring IV nitrates	2
Left ventricular dysfunction	Ejection fraction 30% to 50% Ejection fraction < 30%	1 3
Recent myocardial infarction	< 90 days	2
Pulmonary hypertension	Systolic pulmonary pressure > 60 mm/Hg	2
Emergency operation	Surgery performed on the day of arrival	2
Other than isolated CABG	Addition of any other major cardiac procedure	2
Surgery on thoracic aorta		3
Post myocardial infarction septal rupture		4

Source: Adapted from *Eur. J. Cardiothoracic Surg.* 16:9 (1999): 199.
Note: Low risk: 0–2 points; estimated mortality 1.3%. Medium risk: 3–5 points; estimated mortality 2.9%. High risk: ≥ 6 points; estimated mortality 10.9% to 11.5%.

mortality. The increased risk associated with female gender is probably related to a smaller average body size. Smaller-bodied people usually have smaller coronary arteries and more difficult surgery. Renal (kidney) and neurological functions as well as peripheral vascular status are also significant determinants of mortality risk. Diabetes can adversely affect kidneys and nerves, so the increased risk associated with cardiac surgery in people with diabetes is related to the multisystem involvement of diabetes. Likewise, the adverse impact of smoking is reflected by the presence of chronic obstructive pulmonary disease and pulmonary hypertension. The numbers in table 8.1 reflect the impact of these comorbidities on early postoperative mortality. These conditions strongly influence long-term outcomes following successful cardiac surgery as well.

While there is an essential relationship between the patient's preoperative clinical status and perioperative mortality, there is substantial evidence that who performs the cardiac surgery and where it is performed are incredibly important. Numerous studies have shown that hospitals that perform a low volume of cardiac surgery procedures (generally fewer than 250 procedures per year) have a higher mortality rate than high-volume centers. This difference may not be as apparent for patients considered to be at low risk, but it does seem significant for patients considered to be at medium or high risk for perioperative events. Individual surgeon experience, too, seems to influence perioperative mortality. In the Society of Thoracic Surgeons database, the surgeon's annual caseload inversely correlates with perioperative mortality. Not surprisingly, the highest operative mortality was noted when procedures were performed in low-volume hospitals by low-volume surgeons. Many states now provide online information regarding hospitals' and individual surgeons' experience for cardiac surgery. Don't be shy about asking for information about a surgeon's or hospital's experience in performing coronary bypass surgery. You owe it to yourself to research your purchase of a new coronary blood supply with at least as much diligence as you use in purchasing a new car.

What Are the Potential Complications of Surgery?

Coronary bypass surgery is difficult surgery for even the most experienced and skilled surgeons. Some complications may occur even in the best of hands, and the complications reflect the complexity of the procedure rather than being the fault of any person or place. For example, some degree of blood loss is common following cardiac surgery. Some of the blood loss may represent dilution of the blood by the necessary administration of intravenous fluids during and after surgery. Some of the blood loss may represent the gradual loss of blood from the *resected* (cut) bone and fatty tissues. In the ICU, you will be closely monitored for any blood loss. Life-threatening bleeding following cardiac surgery can occur, but it is uncommon. Only 2 percent of patients need to return to the operating room to control bleeding following surgery. The need for postoperative blood transfusion is somewhat higher, approaching 25 percent of all cases.

Many patients are concerned about blood transfusions, citing the risk of acquiring a blood-borne infection. Today, all blood products are carefully screened for hepatitis and HIV infections. The risk of acquiring these infections from blood transfusion is on the order of one in several million. If your doctor decides that a blood transfusion will speed your recovery, you should consider accepting it. It will make you feel better. Factors that increase your likelihood of requiring a blood transfusion include a low blood count prior to surgery, advancing age, low body weight, and being female. The preoperative use of potent anticoagulants like Coumadin, tissue plasminogen activators, and certain platelet inhibitors all increase the risk of postoperative bleeding. If a patient has been treated with any of these agents, it is customary to delay surgery (if possible) for several days or for the patient to receive a transfusion of coagulation factors to counteract the effects of these agents.

As we saw earlier in this book, aspirin impairs platelet function. With current surgical techniques, the risk of bleeding related to aspirin therapy is no longer thought to be significant, and aspirin is no longer withheld before cardiac surgery. Clopidogrel is another oral platelet inhibitor frequently taken by people with coronary heart disease. Several studies have shown that the preoperative use of clopidogrel is associated with an increased risk for perioperative bleeding. While treatment with clopidogrel may be very beneficial for patients with coronary heart disease, current recommendations suggest that it be discontinued for five days prior to elective cardiac surgery. The difficulty with this recommendation is that many physicians start their patients on clopidogrel before cardiac catheterization, with the intention of performing a percutaneous catheter intervention if the patient needs it (see chapter 7). In these cases, should the patient need cardiac surgery, a delay in surgery is usually prescribed to facilitate the return of platelet function and reduce the risk of postoperative bleeding.

Infection is another postoperative complication that can occur in some patients. A local infection at the site of vein harvesting in the leg may be manifest as a low-grade fever or some localized swelling and inflammation. This type of infection is uncommon, occurring in 3 to 5 percent of patients, and it is usually managed with local wound care and oral antibiotics. The spread of the infection throughout the body is less common. It is generally indicative of an infection somewhere inside the body.

A deep-seated infection of the sternal incision site is much more serious. This life-threatening condition, called *mediastinitis,* is an infection that may extend to the chest below the sternum. Mediastinitis tends to appear seven to ten days after surgery rather than immediately after surgery. The symptoms of this infection are fever, chest pain, and drainage from the sternal incision site. Sometimes there is slight movement and instability of the breastbone. The incidence of mediastinitis is low, averaging less than 1 percent of all surgical procedures. It is a frightening complication and a serious infection that requires prompt and aggressive treatment. Treatment may include surgical *debridement* (surgical removal of necrotic, or dead, tissue) of the infected site and prolonged intravenous antibiotics. Obesity, diabetes, emergency surgery, and the use of both internal mammary arteries in the surgery (discussed later in this chapter) all increase the risk of postoperative mediastinitis.

Many patients fear neurological complications of cardiac surgery more than they fear death. This is understandable given the severe degree of debilitation that neurological injury can produce. The incidence and degree of postoperative neurological dysfunction ranges between 1 and 5 percent of cases, depending on the demographics (age, race, gender) of the patients. Risk factors for postoperative neurological dysfunction include advancing age and being female. Peripheral artery atherosclerotic disease and a history of diabetes, hypertension, or kidney failure are all risk factors for the development of postoperative neurological dysfunction. These problems are clues indicating that the patient may have atherosclerosis of the body's largest vessel, the aorta.

Atherosclerosis of the aorta is the major cause of neurological injury in patients undergoing cardiac surgery. Plate 9 depicts the proximity between the aortic arch, the carotid arteries, and the brain. The inside of an atherosclerotic aortic has the appearance of a cobblestone road. It is covered with atherosclerotic plaque and thrombus that protrude into the lumen of the aorta. Thus, when the aorta is manipulated as a necessary part of any cardiac surgery, plaque may fracture and the debris can be dislodged into the bloodstream. When this debris travels to the brain and obstructs the brain's blood supply, the result is neurological injury.

Neurological injury after cardiac surgery can be divided into two broad categories: injury due to the obstruction of large cerebral vessels (*macrovascular obstruction*) or injury due to the obstruction of small cerebral blood vessels (*microvascular obstruction*). Macrovascular injury is what most people think of when they think of a stroke. Here, obstruction of a large cerebral blood vessel produces focal brain damage that is generally manifested as the inability to move a limb or speak. Microvascular brain injury is much more subtle and can be more difficult to recognize. Here, microscopic debris has been dislodged from the aorta and has traveled through the bloodstream like grains of sand, eventually becoming trapped in microscopic blood vessels. In most places in the body, these microscopic *emboli* produce no symptoms. In the brain, they tend to produce a mild but diffuse injury that can be manifested as some confusion, emotional fragility, or forgetfulness. These nonspecific findings may be most pronounced in the elderly population. The good news about postoperative microvascular injury is that it tends to improve gradually with time. Most patients go on to have a full recovery, approaching their preoperative level of cognitive function.

As noted earlier, the risk for postoperative neurological complication increases with several well-recognized clinical conditions. If you have any of these conditions, your physician may choose to screen you preoperatively for aortic and cerebral atherosclerosis. Screening is commonly done with an ultrasound examination. The *carotid arteries,* which are the blood vessels that supply the brain, are located in the neck (see plate 9). An ultrasound examination of these blood vessels is called a *carotid duplex examination.* (A carotid duplex examination and an echocardiogram—described in chapter 5—are similar in that they both use ultrasound to image structures inside the body, but they use different equipment and look at different structures.) The ultrasound transducer is placed on the neck, directly over the carotid arteries, and an image of these key cerebral vessels is reconstructed by computer. The extent to which these vessels are narrowed by atherosclerotic plaque is readily apparent. Depending on the degree of carotid obstruction present, surgery may be delayed and other tests or treatments ordered.

Imaging of the ascending aorta and aortic arch requires a different type of ultrasound examination. This examination, called a *transesophageal echocardiogram* (TEE), is also different from a transthoracic echocardiogram. The TEE requires putting the patient briefly to sleep, to allow passage of the ultrasound transducer into the esophagus. The esophagus lies directly behind the heart, so imaging from this location eliminates any interference by breast or lung tissue. The resulting images provide excellent views of the aorta and aortic arch. If the TEE identifies atherosclerosis of the aortic arch, the surgeon may be able to modify the surgical techniques to reduce (but not eliminate) the chances of postoperative neurological injury.

Despite the possibility of these complications, coronary bypass surgery is a life-enhancing and life-saving therapeutic alternative. In most patients, it can be performed with a 2 to 5 percent chance of a major complication. Following successful coronary bypass surgery, the overwhelming majority of patients experience a complete relief of their anginal symptoms. For many people, this procedure is truly life saving. If you need a coronary bypass operation, you need to understand its risks and benefits completely. Thoroughly understanding these risks and benefits involves more than just understanding the technical aspects of the surgical procedure. Issues regarding the nature of the coronary bypass grafts and how they are attached have important clinical implications. Living with coronary heart disease means learning about these issues as well.

Different Types of Coronary Bypass Grafts

Take another look at plate 8 and you will see that different types of conduits can be used to create the coronary bypass grafts. While they are all equally effective in providing an alternative blood supply to the heart, they are not all equal in their durability and longevity.

Venous Bypass Grafts

When most people think of coronary bypass surgery, they envision bypass of the blocked artery using a segment of vein harvested from the leg, and venous bypass grafts are certainly the most common—in fact, the most common type of bypass graft is a superficial vein, the *greater saphenous vein,* which is located in the lower leg along the inner ankle and calf. Sometimes a segment of vein is harvested from the upper thigh. In some patients, a considerable length of vein may be harvested from both sites and both legs. The site and extent of harvesting is determined by the surgeon and generally dictated by the quality of the veins and the size of the leg.

The *quality* of the veins is important in determining its suitability to serve as a conduit for a coronary bypass operation. Large, ropelike varicose veins are not well suited for coronary bypass grafts because they may be prone to develop blood clots. But thin, wire-like veins are not ideal, either, because they may not be able to provide the heart with sufficient blood flow. The initial quality of the vein that is used is very important in determining the longevity of the bypass graft. Leg veins may be needed as a graft, so they deserve the very best care all through our lives. If you have a tendency to form varicose veins, you should take efforts to prevent them from getting worse. Wearing support hose will help preserve your leg veins. Most important, do not get the veins of your legs stripped or sclerosed (shriveled) by the injection of materials. Some varicose veins may be suitable for use as coronary bypass grafts. While varicose veins may be somewhat unsightly today, they may be very handy to you if you need bypass surgery in the future.

Saphenous veins have been used as coronary bypass grafts for close to forty years, so a great deal is known about their performance as blood-carrying conduits. One of the most important things to know about saphenous vein grafts is that they do not last forever. *Patency* is the term used to describe an open, freely flowing bypass graft. The likelihood of a bypass being open at a given point in time is referred to as the *patency rate*. Figure 8.1 depicts the patency rate of bypass grafts after successful coronary bypass surgery.

Figure 8.1 indicates that as early as one year after bypass surgery, saphenous vein graft patency is significantly less than 100 percent. That's right: within the first year following surgery, perhaps as many as 10 percent of saphenous vein bypass grafts will close. This early loss may occur within the first days, weeks, or months following surgery. The loss of a bypass graft at this time may not be associated with any new symptoms. At other times, the loss of a saphenous vein graft may be heralded by the return of anginal symptoms or even a heart attack. This variability following early bypass closure occurs because the native coronary artery that was bypassed is usually still open. When the bypass graft closes, flow reverts to the diseased, albeit patent, coronary artery. Patients are sometimes mystified when they find out at the time of a later coronary angiogram that one or several bypass grafts had closed without their knowledge.

Several factors may make early saphenous vein graft loss more likely. Poor vein quality, mentioned above, is very predictive of vein graft loss. Likewise, if the vein is damaged during harvesting from the leg, it may be more likely to close early. Poor coronary artery quality is another clinical consideration. By artery quality, I mean the size of the bypassed coronary artery and its ability to handle increased coronary blood flow. Ideally, the coronary bypass graft completely circumvents the area of atherosclerotic disease, allowing the downstream portion

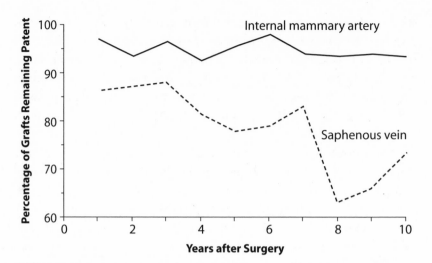

FIGURE 8.1. Coronary bypass graft patency ten years after surgery. This figure depicts the patency (that is, the likelihood of remaining open) in internal mammary vein bypass grafts and saphenous vein bypass grafts. Note how after the first year following surgery, internal mammary graft patency remains constant at about 95 percent. Saphenous vein grafts, however, continue to have falling patency rates. This difference in bypass graft patency rates is directly attributable to the viable endothelial layer present in internal mammary artery bypass grafts. (Adapted from F. D. Loop, "Influence of the Internal-Mammary-Artery Graft on 10-Year Survival and Other Cardiac Events," *New England Journal of Medicine* 314 (1986): 1–6.)

of the bypass graft to be inserted into a reasonably normal segment of the artery.

Picture the bypass conduit's two ends. One is the beginning of the bypass graft, where it is attached to the aorta. The other, so-called downstream segment of the graft, is the segment that is attached to the coronary artery in the heart. The medical terms are *proximal anastomosis* (at the aorta) and *distal anastomosis* (the downstream portion).

If the downstream arterial segment is very small or if the coronary artery has diffuse atherosclerotic disease, the flow through the bypass graft will be slow. This slow flow in the bypass graft will make it more likely to develop thrombus and ultimately to occlude. The amount of flow through the bypass graft and its downstream "runoff" is crucial for maintaining early bypass graft patency. You can imagine that having many downstream connections will increase the flow through one bypass graft, and sometimes a surgeon will use the same saphenous vein to make many downstream anastomoses in an attempt to increase the overall flow through the bypass graft. This type of coronary bypass graft is referred to as a *jump graft,* or *sequential bypass graft.* The number of downstream anastomoses that can be done is limited by the amount of suitable vein available, the number of suitable coronary artery segments where the bypass graft can be attached, and the duration of surgery.

It usually doesn't make sense to bypass minimally diseased coronary arteries, because there is a significant relationship between high coronary bypass flow and graft patency. Unless there is significant atherosclerotic narrowing, flow through the native coronary artery will be quite good. If this minimally diseased coronary artery is bypassed, the bypass graft may carry very little blood flow and, with minimal blood flow, the bypass graft will eventually *thrombose* (become blocked by a thrombus). Bypassing minimally diseased coronary arteries now, "just in case" they narrow or thrombose, is not useful.

Early graft thrombosis is a serious problem following successful coronary bypass surgery. Much of the early clotting of saphenous vein grafts is begun by platelet aggregation. Inhibiting platelet function helps minimize the chance of early vein graft thrombosis. All patients who undergo coronary bypass surgery are started on aspirin and clopidogrel, potent inhibitors of platelet function, very early in the postoperative period. Taking this step has been shown to significantly improve early bypass graft patency, and beyond that, there is benefit in patients who have bypass surgery taking these medications for the rest of their lives, because the risk of platelet aggregation and graft thrombosis persists. Figure 8.1 reveals that early graft patency is not the only challenge facing patients with successful coronary bypass graft surgery. Even if a saphenous vein remains patent for the first year after surgery, there is an ongoing tendency for the bypass graft to occlude each year thereafter. The risk of losing a bypass graft is about 1 to 3 percent each year and accumulates throughout the life of the graft so that ten years after successful coronary bypass surgery, the saphenous vein graft patency rate is only about 70 to 80 percent. The cause of this late bypass graft loss is different from the cause of early graft loss.

When harvesting a vein from the leg, the surgeon excises it (cuts it) from the body. Its microscopic nerve and vascular supply are disrupted, and so, in essence, it no longer serves as living tissue. As a bypass graft, the saphenous vein essentially functions like an inert hose, simply carrying blood around the blocked coronary artery. It sits there, physiologically inactive. It can't dilate to increase its flow in response to metabolic demands; nor can it constrict to maintain its blood pressure and flow if the person's blood pressure gets low. This lack of physiological response is distinctly different from the active response of an artery and is due to malfunction in the vein graft's endothelial lining. Excised saphenous veins produce much less nitric oxide and are far less vasoreactive than veins that are left in place. The excised and dysfunctional saphenous vein also fails to produce several other endothelial-derived substances that normally prevent thrombosis and inflammation.

As a result of all these factors, saphenous vein grafts are not only prone to produce thromboses, they are also susceptible to a rapid growth of atheroscleroticlike material inside the graft. Aging saphenous veins can go on and produce flow-limiting narrowings at a rate that is much faster than the rate in native coronary arteries. These bypass graft stenoses ultimately clot, and the clots make their presence known by the return of angina or a heart attack some years after successful bypass surgery.

The situation with later bypass graft closure is distinctly different than with early bypass graft closure. In fact, it is the exact opposite. When there is high blood flow through the bypass graft, blood flow through the diseased native coronary artery falls, predisposing it to thrombus formation. When there is a normally functioning coronary bypass graft, this progression in the native coronary artery occurs silently, without any symptoms. In this setting, the development of any narrowing of the bypass graft now takes on a special significance, because the native coronary artery is not useful. The bypass graft is the primary conduit of blood for a portion of the heart, and any reduction in its flow is usually heralded by the return of anginal symptoms.

The gradual development of bypass graft stenosis is an almost inevitable aftereffect of coronary bypass surgery. Sometimes it happens fairly soon after the procedure. Other times it occurs many years later. When it does happen, many patients feel as if they have done something wrong. This is generally not the case. The development of late bypass graft loss is a manifestation of *aging and deterioration of the graft*. The progressive deterioration of saphenous vein grafts is ubiquitous and difficult to prevent.

Attempts to prevent and treat *bypass graft disease* have not been very rewarding. Platelet inhibition with aspirin and suppression of circulating LDL with high-dose statin agents provides some help, and many patients are started on these medications within the first few days after coronary bypass surgery. Beta-blocking agents, angiotensin-converting enzyme (ACE) inhibitors, and even fish oils have all been tried, without much success. The bypass graft form of atherosclerotic disease is very resistant to most forms of treatment. Smoking, kidney failure, and diabetes all seem to increase the risk of developing vein graft narrowings, and these conditions must be carefully managed (and smoking stopped) after any coronary bypass procedure.

Bypass graft disease is more like the accumulation of leaves inside a rain gutter than it is like the atherosclerosis described in chapter 2. Once a saphenous vein graft narrowing develops, it is difficult to treat. Angioplasty and stent deployment in an aging bypass graft is more difficult and riskier than it is in a native coronary artery. This is because of the large amounts of debris that tend to accumulate within the bypass graft. Manipulation of the bypass graft with the angioplasty balloon or stent may cause this debris to dislodge and travel downstream to the heart, where it may completely disrupt coronary blood flow and cause a heart attack. As a result, PCI of vein grafts has been associated with a higher risk of complications and a higher mortality than PCI of a native coronary artery. Some intravascular filters may be used to minimize but not eliminate this risk of debris dislodgment. Even with drug-eluting stents, the suppression of the hyperproliferative response and accumulation of debris within the aging vein graft has not been great. In fact, some reports suggest that in aging saphenous vein grafts, drug-eluting stents may not necessarily be superior to bare metal stents.

Fixing one stenosis in an aging bypass graft is usually not the end of the story. The deterioration of these grafts represents a process that extends throughout the conduit, and therefore these aggressive narrowings tend to recur, if not within the stented segment, then elsewhere in the degenerating vein graft. Not surprisingly, many patients who undergo PCI in an aging saphenous vein graft later undergo an additional PCI procedure at another location. The detection of a stenosis in an aging saphenous vein bypass graft is like noting that the bathroom wallpaper has started to peel away in one location. You may fix one patch, but you know it will soon begin to peel away in other places. For this reason, some patients undergo a repeat coronary bypass operation when multiple aged bypass grafts are narrowed, if the operation is technically feasible and the patient's overall health is good.

A repeat coronary bypass operation is more challenging and riskier than the initial coronary bypass procedure. Not only is the patient older than he or she was at the time of the initial coronary bypass operation, the patient may be sicker due to progression of other medical problems such as diabetes, kidney failure, and chronic obstructive pulmonary disease. For a repeat coronary bypass operation, suitable veins must be found to serve as bypass conduits, when large sections of the most suitable veins may already have been harvested at the time of the original bypass procedure. To perform the second bypass operation, the surgeon needs to navigate through the earlier sternal incision and scar tissue that is invariably present in the area of the operation.

Not surprisingly, a repeat coronary bypass operation generally has a perioperative complication and mortality rate that is two to three times greater than the rate of the initial procedure. In most patients there is about a 4 to 8 percent chance of a major complication. For all these reasons, some patients may be reluctant to undergo a second coronary bypass operation. A second coronary bypass procedure can, however, provide patients with an extended symptom-free period. Many patients who have "redo" coronary bypass surgery go on to live long and healthy lives. There is nothing to suggest that a person who experiences premature degeneration of the first set of coronary bypass grafts will have a similar outcome with the second set. In people with multivessel coronary artery stenoses, compromised ventricular function, or diabetes mellitus, a coronary bypass procedure, either initially or as a redo, remains the procedure of choice for improving both the quality and the quantity of life.

Arterial Bypass Grafts

In some cases there is an alternative to using saphenous veins for coronary bypass graft. Under the right circumstances, there is a possibility of using the *internal mammary artery* (IMA) as a bypass conduit. (Sometimes this artery is referred to as the *internal thoracic artery.*) There are two IMAs located beneath the chest wall just to the right (RIMA) and left (LIMA) of the sternum. These arteries supply blood to the sternal area and muscles between the ribs. These structures have a dual blood supply, meaning that a person can do just fine without one internal mammary artery. If one IMA is missing, nearby blood vessels appear to be capable of supplying blood to adjacent tissues. This redundancy of the IMA has opened the possibility for its use as a bypass conduit, and the IMA has several distinct advantages over the saphenous vein for this purpose.

In the field of coronary bypass surgery, there was some initial concern that the IMA was too small to serve as an effective conduit for the myocardial blood supply. Furthermore, its location beneath the chest wall made it technically difficult to harvest. The additional surgery certainly increased the risk of postoperative bleeding and infection. This slight increase in operative risk, however, is more than offset by the long-term benefit of using this vessel as a bypass conduit. As figure 8.1 clearly shows, the internal mammary artery has a significant patency advantage over the saphenous vein graft. Far fewer grafts are lost in the first year following surgery, and the ten-year patency is 97 percent.

As with the saphenous vein graft, some internal mammary artery grafts appear to close in the first year, but to a lesser degree. There are several reasons for this closure. Early loss of the IMA graft is generally attributed to scar tissue formation at the site of the downstream anastomosis with the native coronary artery. Some early graft loss may be due to diffuse downstream disease of the native coronary artery, so that adequate flow never develops in the IMA graft, or the graft may have been used to bypass a minimally diseased artery (as discussed above). Nonetheless, there are fairly good one-year patency rates for IMA grafts. More important than this short-term patency are the excellent long-term results. An IMA graft that is patent at one year after surgery tends to stay open for a very long time. Why is there such a striking difference in long-term patency between the internal mammary artery and saphenous vein grafts? Once again, the answer involves the all-important endothelial lining of the blood vessel.

Unlike a saphenous vein, the internal mammary artery is a bona fide artery. It is built to handle pressurized blood flow. It has well-developed adventitia, media, and endothelial layers. Structurally, it is just like the normal segment of coronary artery depicted in plate 2A. The IMA is functionally similar to a coronary artery, too, because to be used as a coronary bypass conduit, the IMA need not be completely excised from its native location and reimplanted. This means that it is alive and functioning. In plate 8 you can see that one end of the internal mammary artery remains intact and attached to its parent blood vessel. The microscopic nerve and vascular supply to the artery also remains intact and adherent to the blood vessel. Notice that the internal mammary is encased in a vascular *pedicle* containing these structures. The pedicle is the residual tissue surrounding a blood vessel. Its continued association with these structures enables the internal mammary to remain alive and vasoreactive. The vascular endothelium of the IMA graft remains functional and produces all the protective substances that help retard the formation of thrombus and atherosclerosis. In many ways, using the IMA graft as a bypass conduit is like giving the patient a brand new coronary artery. Its use, when technically feasible, has become standard in coronary bypass surgery.

Patient outcome data clearly demonstrate that the revascularization procedures utilizing the LIMA as a bypass graft provide superior long-term outcomes than those that do not. Unfortunately, there are limitations to the use of the internal mammary artery in coronary bypass surgery. The LIMA is most frequently used as a bypass conduit to the left anterior descending coronary artery (LAD). This is because of its proximity to the front of the heart and the location of the LAD, just below the sternum. Because one end of the LIMA must remain attached to the aorta near its origin at the base of the neck, the surgeon can use only so much length of internal mammary artery to reach the heart. It is difficult, if not impossible, to have the LIMA extend to other coronary arteries on the side or back of the heart. In women with low body weight or small stature or in elderly people, the LIMA may be too small and thus cannot be used as a bypass conduit. Excising the LIMA from is origin and using it as a free bypass graft significantly reduces its viability as a bypass vessel. Despite these limitations, the LIMA is now used as the bypass graft to the LAD in over 90 percent of coronary bypass procedures. It is unquestionably an excellent bypass conduit that provides patients with a durable blood supply.

Many patients ask, if using one internal mammary artery is good, wouldn't using two internal mammary arteries be better? After all, there are left and right internal mammary arteries. Considering the length limitations imposed by using the LIMA as a bypass graft, we can understand that the RIMA, which resides in the right chest wall, is a long way from the heart, which is located in the left chest. Nonetheless, the RIMA can be used in certain situations as a coronary bypass graft. It is generally used to bypass narrowings in the right coronary artery (and sometimes the left circumflex artery), which resides on the back of the heart and hence lies closest to the right chest. While the RIMA is an excellent bypass conduit, its use poses some significant technical challenges.

The combined use of the LIMA and RIMA is unquestionably a more complicated and riskier surgical procedure than use of a single IMA. Plate 9 depicts the location of the IMAs prior to their use as bypass conduits. Isolating both vessels requires surgical dissections inside both the left and right chest walls. This creates a longer surgical procedure, a longer postoperative stay in the intensive care unit, and a higher incidence of postoperative bleeding. Branches of the internal mammary arteries provide the blood supply to the sternum and ribs. The combined use of the LIMA and the RIMA can also compromise the blood supply to the area of the sternal incision. The use of both internal mammary arteries removes some of the capacity for redundancy in supplying blood to adjacent tissues that was discussed earlier. Not surprisingly, coronary bypass surgery that uses both internal mammary arteries is associated with an increased risk of inadequate sternal healing and chest wall infections. This is particularly true in people with diabetes, who tend to have small arteries and an impaired ability to fight infection. As a result of these limitations, both mammary arteries are not routinely used in coronary bypass surgery. Nonetheless, in some selected patients, the combined use of the LIMA and RIMA makes sense. Long-term results with these bypass grafts are very favorable with respect to mortality, return of angina, and the need for a repeat revascularization. Your surgeon will decide what type of bypass graft is best for you depending on your size, age, general health, and other factors.

An artery unquestionably has many attractive features that favor its uses as a bypass conduit. Unfortunately, not many arteries are as easily expendable as the internal mammary artery. One possible candidate is the radial artery. The radial artery supplies the hand with blood. It is the artery in the wrist that is frequently felt when taking your pulse. The hand has the good fortune of having a dual blood supply, and hence the radial artery can be excised without any compromise in the blood supply to the hand. There has been considerable interest in using the radial artery as an alternative to the saphenous vein graft. Unlike the internal mammary artery, the radial artery is excised from its native location and used as a free graft to bypass a blocked coronary artery.

As an arterial conduit with fully developed media and endothelial layers, the radial artery has some theoretical advantages over the saphenous vein grafts. The long-term results of coronary bypass procedures using this vessel in bypass grafts have been mixed, however. Several large surgical centers have reported favorable patency rates using the radial artery while others have reported an excessive rate of early closure. This closure rate has been attributed to the small caliber of the radial artery and the vessel's susceptibility to develop spasm, as well as its relative fragility and tendency to be damaged during the harvesting procedure. As a result, some centers have abandoned its use as a bypass conduit. The Radial Artery Patency Study (RAPS) is an international, multicenter study examining the role of the radial artery in patients with coronary bypass surgery. The most recent results from the RAPS group suggest that the radial artery may be superior to the saphenous vein graft in some well-defined circumstances. Follow-up from RAPS has been limited to only one year, and the number of patients studied is relatively small.

Experience with the radial artery as a bypass graft is continually being accumulated, and the role of this artery in coronary bypass procedures continues to evolve. Current surgical practice, however, dictates that the LIMA is the initial conduit of choice for coronary bypass grafting. The RIMA is equally suitable when double-vessel coronary bypass grafting is clinically indicated and when its use is technically feasible. The saphenous vein or radial artery is a third alternative for conduits in patients who may require multivessel bypass grafts. In emergency or difficult surgical situations, usually the saphenous vein, and not the internal mammary artery, is used for the sake of expediency.

Coronary stent procedures are increasing in number and success, but a coronary bypass operation remains a very effective form of treatment in the right patients and in the right circumstances, providing nearly all patients with complete relief of their angina symptoms. In patients who receive a complete revascularization, the left ventricle may exhibit a significant improvement in contractile function and therefore improve long-term prognosis. Following coronary bypass surgery, many patients are able to return to work and resume normal and productive lives. The greatest limitation to coronary bypass surgery is that it is highly invasive and involves an extended convalescence period. In recent years, improvements in surgical techniques have had significant effects in both these areas.

New and Emerging Coronary Bypass Procedures

As described early in this chapter, cardiac surgery involves stopping the heart and turning the duties of circulatory support and oxygenation of tissue over to an external machine. The need for cardiopulmonary bypass significantly complicates the surgery, because the aorta must be manually manipulated, or *cross-clamped*. This procedure creates a risk of dislodging aortic debris, causing a stroke. In addition, in some patients, there is evidence that passage of the blood through the cardiopulmonary bypass machine may produce an inflammatory state that may contribute to some of the neurological and pulmonary changes that are sometimes seen in the postoperative period. For these reasons and more, some centers perform coronary bypass surgery without the use of cardiopulmonary bypass. This type of surgery is frequently referred to as OP-CABG, for *off-pump coronary artery bypass grafting*.

OP-CABG is technically more difficult than traditional coronary bypass grafting. With the heart still beating, the surgeon must sew the small coronary bypass grafts to a moving heart. Sewing on a moving target is made possible by using specialized equipment during surgery to stabilize and reduce the motion of the heart. Since the heart is still beating, and thus responsible for supporting the body's circulation, manipulation of the beating heart to sew the bypass grafts may produce significant changes in blood pressure or cardiac rhythm. The patient's underlying condition is a large factor in determining whether the patient is a candidate for OP-CABG. Not everyone is.

There is a steep learning curve to performing successful OP-CABG, and not all surgeons can perform this procedure equally well. The use of OP-CABG varies among surgical centers from as few as 10 percent of all procedures to over 90 percent. The greatest benefit of OP-CABG is in the avoidance of cardiopulmonary bypass and all its complications. In experienced hands, OP-CABG is associated with a decreased incidence of neurological complications, preservation of kidney function, and a shorter hospital stay. Because bypass grafts are sewn onto a beating heart, there has always been some concern regarding the formation of stricture at the anastomosis with the native coronary artery and the long-term patency of the bypass grafts, but centers with experience performing large numbers of these procedures have reported bypass graft patency rates that are comparable to those of traditional bypass surgery.

The eventual role of OP-CABG in treating patients with coronary heart disease is yet to be defined. For now its greatest benefit seems to be in elderly people with severely atherosclerotic aortas, where the risk of neurological complications from aortic cross-clamping is high. It may also have a role in certain high-risk procedures where stopping the heart to institute full cardiopulmonary bypass support is deemed too risky. Off-pump CABG may also be useful in patients who do not need multivessel coronary bypass grafts. In these patients, the OP-CABG technique may facilitate a less invasive bypass procedure and quicker recuperation.

Both OP-CABG and traditional coronary bypass surgery require trans-sectioning of the sternal bone, so they are considered highly invasive surgeries. Sternal incision is the major source of discomfort and morbidity in the postoperative period. In patients who require a bypass of only one coronary artery, a less invasive approach may be practical. This is frequently referred to as *minimally invasive coronary artery bypass grafting* (MID-CABG). A MID-CABG surgical procedure is generally performed through a much smaller surgical incision, between the ribs. Sometimes this type of coronary bypass surgery is referred to as *keyhole surgery* because of the shape of the incision.

In MID-CABG the surgical field is much smaller and multiple vessels cannot be bypassed through a single incision. The MID-CABG technique can be used with or without cardiopulmonary bypass, but the majority of MID-CABG procedures are performed without cardiopulmonary bypass support. If needed, cardiopulmonary bypass can be instituted via access to the large femoral arteries and veins located in the groin. By avoiding a large sternal incision, the MID-CABG procedure generally produces a more rapid recovery than traditional surgery does. A MID-CABG procedure, because it avoids a sternal incision, may have a useful role when redo coronary bypass surgery is needed or in certain high-risk scenarios.

The concept of a MID-CABG, or keyhole, procedure can be extended to surgery performed through multiple smaller incisions using fiberoptic scopes and computer-assisted robotics. This type of minimally invasive robotic surgery is available at an increasing number of surgical centers in the United States and abroad. The small robotic arms facilitate surgery within a closed chest. Mechanically guided and computer assisted, these robotic arms have the potential for allowing the surgeon to perform very delicate and accurate maneuvers in a small space. The collective experience with this robotic technique is fairly small, and long-term patient outcomes are unavailable. Nonetheless, this is exciting technology that will unquestionably evolve with time.

For now, robot-assisted coronary bypass grafting must be considered a niche procedure performed by highly trained surgeons in carefully selected patients.

We return now to James, who had a markedly abnormal stress test. His coronary angiogram had confirmed that he has triple-vessel coronary artery disease with a moderate degree of left ventricular damage. A coronary revascularization was unquestionably the procedure of choice, and James and his doctor decided to proceed with traditional coronary bypass grafting, via a midline sternal incision.

After tests to further evaluate his operative candidacy, James had triple-vessel coronary bypass surgery. His doctors estimated his risk for major complications, including death, to be 2 percent. At the time of surgery, James received a LIMA graft to the left anterior descending coronary artery, a RIMA graft to the right coronary artery, and a saphenous vein graft to the left circumflex artery. He did very well. Aside from some transient atrial fibrillation on postoperative day three, James had no postoperative complications. He was discharged on the sixth postoperative day. His medications were aspirin, clopidogrel, a beta-blocking drug, a statin agent, and a mild diuretic. He was scheduled to see his doctor in two weeks.

James's immediate problem has been addressed, but his need to prevent and treat atherosclerosis will go on for the rest of his life. He is taking many different medications, despite his initial reluctance, and each one is designed to attack a specific component of the atherosclerotic process. Yet, eventually, James found out that living with coronary heart disease can mean living a normal, productive, and active life even after surgery. It's time to find out how.

NINE

Living with Coronary Heart Disease

J ames was anxious to get home, take a shower, and sleep in his own bed. The first few nights at home were a bit rocky, however. Like many people who have had heart surgery, James had trouble sleeping at first. What had transpired in the past two weeks could overwhelm anyone. Emotions run high, and many people feel blue.

As noted in chapter 8, bypass surgery is major surgery, and recovery takes time. In this chapter, we will discuss patients' most common concerns in the weeks and months right after surgery, and then look at how people can live confidently with coronary heart disease.

After Surgery

Some people are concerned about the strength of the sternal incision. The incision is actually very durable and will hold up well during the activities of everyday living, although care must be taken until the sternum is fully fused. (This generally takes about four weeks.) During this time, avoid doing any heavy lifting or activities that may cause the breastbone to twist, such as driving a car.

Some postoperative soreness is common and may be relieved with a mild analgesic for a few days at home. Ask your doctor what you should take to relieve pain. The need for prescription painkillers is minimal, generally for no longer than a week or two following surgery. Any sternal discomfort that continues longer than two weeks requires investigation by your doctor.

The stress of surgery significantly activates your sympathetic nervous system, and as we saw in chapter 6, this fight-or-flight response releases a great deal of epinephrine into your bloodstream. Because of this stress, after surgery many people have a rapid or irregular heartbeat and will be discharged from the hospital with a beta-blocking agent to help keep the heart rate slow and the rhythm regular.

Some people may experience a loss of appetite and disruption of bowel habits for several days following coronary bypass surgery, and it is not uncommon to lose five to ten pounds after surgery. Your appetite will return, and your bodily functions will soon be back to normal.

Once you are at home, you may find that well-intentioned loved ones bring you plates bearing fish, chicken, and salads—and this is a good thing, since most people with coronary heart disease need to modify their diet, and these foods are heart-healthy foods. Diet is part of a long-term effort to modify cardiovascular risk factors and adopt a healthy lifestyle. In the first few weeks following open-heart surgery, it is essential to try to eat, both to regain your strength and to maintain an adequate level of hydration. Ask your doctor about any dietary restrictions you may have.

Here are some other dos and don'ts for the first few weeks after surgery.

- Follow your doctor's instructions and take your prescribed medications. Ask your doctor how you can reach him or her in case you have any questions. Surgeons' assistants will answer questions they feel comfortable answering, and they also know when it's better for the patient to speak directly to the surgeon.

- Go for light walks daily to improve your appetite and general sense of well-being. While day-to-day improvements may seem minimal, week-to-week progress will be evident.

- Make every effort to keep sternal and other surgical incisions dry. A shower or quick bath is acceptable. Incisions usually require minimal care. Inspect them every day for any signs of redness or drainage. Notify your doctor of any change in their appearance.

- Continue to work on the breathing exercises you were taught while you were in the hospital. These exercises will fully expand your lungs, enable you to breathe more easily, and minimize any chance of developing pneumonia.

- Report to your doctor if you have a *persistent* cough. A mild cough is not uncommon following surgery.

- Wear support hose to minimize any mild swelling of the feet. This is usually more pronounced in the leg from which the saphenous veins were harvested. Your doctor may prescribe a mild diuretic to assist in eliminating some of the excess postoperative fluid retention.

Reducing Your Risks

Whether you have had heart surgery or not, if you have coronary heart disease, you need to take all the steps described in this book to protect your heart's health. Taking steps to control coronary heart disease is essential whether you had coronary bypass surgery, a percutaneous catheter intervention, or none of these procedures but have experienced angina symptoms. Any type of revascularization procedure is really only a plumbing solution, because coronary heart disease is a chronic systemic disorder that requires ongoing suppression of platelets, inflammation, and cholesterol production. Living with coronary heart disease means continually monitoring the risk factors for the disease and taking measures to reduce your risks as well as you are able.

Nearly everyone with coronary heart disease must take medications to inhibit platelet aggregation and platelet activation (see chapter 5), so unless there is a strong contraindication, you will take aspirin and possibly clopidogrel daily. Most people with coronary heart disease also take a statin. If you have had surgery, you will probably start taking a statin as soon as your dietary pattern has normalized, if not sooner. Your doctor will prescribe other medications if they are appropriate for you.

Smoking is no longer an option. *You must stop smoking.*

If you have a history of high blood pressure, the high blood pressure may not be apparent in the early postoperative period, but unfortunately, it may return as your diet and level of activity improves.

Your doctor will be vigilant in monitoring you for high blood pressure and will treat it aggressively if you develop it.

Many people with diabetes find it difficult to control their glucose levels soon after surgery. For some people, weight reduction and improved dietary habits will bring the levels under control. In others, aggressive treatment with one or more medications will be in order. *The importance of strict diabetic management cannot be overstated.* Uncontrolled diabetes can make the treatment of coronary heart disease very difficult.

The American Heart Association (www.americanheart.org) is a source of much valuable information about nutrition, exercise, medications, and many other issues that you need to know about.

Your doctor and your family and friends can help you as much as you need them to help you and as much as you will allow them to help you. If you are a person who does best in a structured, scheduled program, however, then enrolling in a cardiac rehabilitation program may be a wonderful boost for your efforts to stay healthy.

Cardiac Rehabilitation Programs

James returned to his doctor two weeks after surgery. He was eating and sleeping well. He was much less sore than he had been. While anxious to return to work, he also understood the need for some restraint. After meeting with his doctor, James agreed that the best way to ensure his long-term well-being was to enroll in a cardiac rehabilitation program.

Cardiac rehabilitation programs take many forms. They usually involve a supervised exercise program, which may or may not include electrocardiographic monitoring. In addition to helping people develop the confidence and discipline to participate in regular exercise, cardiac rehabilitation programs offer a continuous source of nutrition counseling and encouragement. They provide emotional support and encouragement to stop smoking and not start smoking again. They assist your physician in monitoring your blood pressure and cardiovascular risk factors. For many people, a cardiac rehabilitation program provides much-needed motivation and direction in establishing a healthy lifestyle.

Turning Back the Clock

People with coronary heart disease sometimes worry that "the damage has already been done, so what's the use of trying?" Or they may think, "I'm too old and set in my ways to make lifestyle changes now." Nothing could be further from the truth. It's never too late, and you are never too old to adopt a healthy lifestyle. Consider a study published in 2007 aptly called "Turning Back the Clock: Adopting a Healthy Lifestyle in Middle Age." This study reviewed the impact of lifestyle modification in 15,792 Americans between the ages of 45 and 64. It found that regardless of age, adopting four key lifestyle modifications reduces the risk of developing cardiovascular disease by 35 percent and reduces the chances of dying by 40 percent in as little as four years. The lifestyle modifications associated with this improvement in prognosis were

- eating five fruits and vegetables every day;
- engaging in light exercise for two and a half hours per week;
- maintaining a stable body weight with a body mass index (BMI) between 18.5 and 30 (you can find BMI calculators on the Internet, including on the American Heart Association web site); and
- complete smoking cessation.

Unfortunately, only 8.5 percent of the study population adopted all four lifestyle changes. Smoking cessation is clearly the most difficult lifestyle change to achieve; for many people, smoking is more than a habit, it's an addiction. Your doctor can help you find a program to quit smoking that will work for you. In addition to nicotine withdrawal methods (nicotine patches, gum, or spray), various medications can help reduce the cravings and mood swings that may accompany nicotine withdrawal. Smoking cessation can be achieved, but it takes a strong commitment from the patient and his or her family and friends.

The dramatic results of the Turning Back the Clock Study serve as encouragement for everyone to adopt a healthy lifestyle to prevent or control atherosclerosis. If you have coronary heart disease, it's never too late to adopt a healthy lifestyle and significantly improve your cardiovascular health. Like James, you should start today.

After four weeks of convalescence at home, James returned to full and unrestricted activities. He enrolled in a cardiac rehabilitation program, intent on protecting his most valuable asset: his cardiovascular health. Trim and fit, James is enjoying his new lease on life. Like you, he has become a student of coronary heart disease. He keeps well informed about the new and evolving diagnostic and therapeutic options. He now sees his doctor regularly and monitors his medications and his success in modifying his atherosclerotic risk factors. With his doctor's help, he is able to fully participate in the decision-making process that will affect his health. Like you, he is confident, committed, and fully capable of living with coronary heart disease.

Index

Atherosclerotic process, 6–7, 11–12, 14, 16–17, 28
Atorvastatin (Lipitor), **35**, 92
Atrial fibrillation, 156
Avapro (irbesartan), **123**

Balloon surgery. *See* Coronary angioplasty
Bayesian analysis, 60
Benazepril (Lotensin), **123**
Benicar (olmesartan), **123**
Beta Blocker Heart Attack Trial (BHAT), 110–12
Beta-blocking drugs, 2, 66, 109–12, **110**, **111**, 118, 178; for bypass graft disease, 169; combining with alpha blockers, 113–15; to reduce repeat heart attack risk, 110–12, **111**
Beta receptors, 107–8
Betaxolol (Kerlone), **110**
Bextra (valdecoxib), 88
Bile acids, 9, 10, 33–34
Bisoprolol (Zebeta), **110**
Bleeding: after coronary bypass surgery, 160; intracranial, 147; PCI and, 147
Blocadren (timolol), **110**
Blood-borne infections, 160
Blood clot–dissolving drugs, 145–47, **146**
Blood clotting: as coronary angioplasty complication, 132; coronary artery occlusion due to, 23–24, 86; in diabetes, 48; due to cardiac remodeling, 27–28; estrogen and, 45; hs-CRP and, 40; medications for prevention of, 40, 85–91; smoking and, 53; on stent, 137
Blood glucose control, 47–49, 182
Blood pressure: high (*see* Hypertension); kidney function and, 120–21
Blood transfusion, 160
Body mass index (BMI), 53–54, 183
Bradykinins, **122**, 124–25
Brain damage after cardiac surgery, 162–63
Breathing exercises after surgery, 156, 180–81
Bruce protocol, 65, **65**
Bypass graft disease, 169–70

Calan (verapamil), **117**
Calcium, 62, 115–16
Calcium-channel-blocking drugs, 115–19, **117**
Calcium score, 62
cAMP, 107
Candesartan (Atacand), **123**
Capoten (captopril), **123**
CAPRICORN study, 114–15
Captopril (Capoten), **123**
Cardene (nicardipine), **117**
Cardiac anesthesiologist, 153
Cardiac catheterization, 2, 78–80, 127
Cardiac muscle: damaged portions of, 26, 27; hypertrophy of, 27; infarct expansion of, 27
Cardiac rehabilitation, 182–83
Cardiac remodeling, 27, 124
Cardiac scar tissue, 26–27
Cardif (nitrendipine), **117**
Cardioplegia, 154, 155
Cardiopulmonary bypass (CPB) machine, 154, 155, 175–76
Cardiovascular diseases, 3–4, **4**, **5**
Cardizem (diltiazem), **117**
Cardura (doxazosin), 113
Carotid arteries, 163
Carotid duplex examination, 163
Carvedilol (Coreg), **110**, 114–15
Catapres (clonidine), 112
Celecoxib (Celebrex), 88
Cell surface receptors, 106–7, 114
Cerivastatin, 93
cGMP, 101–3, 107
Chest discomfort, 1, 18, 57–61; during stress test, 66, 68
Chest x-ray, 61
Cholesterol, 8–11; autoregulation of, 9–10; "bad," 11, 35 (*see also* Low density lipoprotein); CHD and, 16, 30–38; in diet, 10, 30–31, 97; functions of, 8–9; "good," 36 (*see also* High density lipoprotein); liver's production of, 34–35
Cholesterol-lowering medications, 33–34, 91–98; cholestyramine, 33–34, 97; ezetimibe, 97; fibrates, 37, 48, 95–96; niacin, 36–37, 96; statins, 2, 34–35, **35**, 40–41, 48, 92–94

Cholesteryl ester transfer protein (CETP), 37, 48; inhibitors of, 37–38
Cholestyramine (Questran), 33–34, 97
Chylomicrons, 10–11
Cialis (tadalafil), 102
Clinical Outcomes Utilizing Revascularization and Aggressive Drug Evaluation (COURAGE) trial, 138–39
Clinical research trials, 31–33
Clogged arteries. *See* Atherosclerotic plaque
Clonidine (Catapres), 112
Clopidogrel (Plavix), 90–91, 178, 181; for angioplasty with stenting, 133, 137; for coronary bypass surgery, 167; preoperative use of, 160–61
Clopidogrel versus Aspirin in Patients at Risk for Ischemic Events (CAPRIE) trial, 90–91
Clot-busting drugs, 145–47, **146**
Collateral arteries, 81–82, 152
Congestive heart failure, 27, 28, 114, 118, 124, 156; alpha- and beta-blocking drugs for, 114–15
Coreg (carvedilol), **110**, 114–15
Corgard (nadolol), **110**
Coronary angioplasty, 2, 127, 130–33; in aging saphenous vein graft, 169; *vs.* medications, 138–40; restenosis after, 133–36; with stenting, 133–38; success of, 132–33, 136
Coronary angioscopy, 138
Coronary arteries, 4–5; anastomosis between bypass graft and, 154–55; arteriosclerotic process in walls of, **6**, 11–12; assessing blood flow in, 69–76, **73**; endothelial lining of, 13–14; layers of, 12–13; normal function of, 12; number of diseased, 128–29; occlusion of, by atherosclerotic plaque, 23–26; remodeling of, 16, 17; spasm of, 57, 117; stenosis of, 81, 117; vasodilator response of, 19
Coronary arteriography, 77–84, **79**, 127–28; benefits and limitations of, 81; cardiac catheterization for, 78–80; complications of, 82–84, **82**; contrast agent for, 78–79, 83–84; indications for, 83, **84**; interpretation of, 128

Coronary artery bypass grafting (CABG), 140. *See also* Coronary bypass surgery
Coronary Artery Surgery Study (CASS), 129
Coronary brachytherapy, 133
Coronary bypass surgery, 2, 130, 132, 134, 139; arterial bypass grafts in, 171–75; complications of, 160–64; hospital's and surgeon's experience with, 159; indications for, 151–52; minimally invasive, 177; new and emerging procedures for, 175–78; number of vessels bypassed in, 155; off-pump, 176–77; outcome of, 175; *vs.* PCI, 140–44, 150; procedure for, 152–57; recovery from, 155–57; risks of, 157–59, **158**; robot-assisted, 177–78; venous bypass grafts in, 164–71, **166**; what to expect after, 179–81
Coronary heart disease (CHD), 4; cholesterol and, 16, 30–38; diabetes and, 47–51; hypertension and, 51–52; invasion of blood vessel wall by, 11–12; medications for, 2, 12, 85–126; mortality from, 4, **5**, 128–29; PCI for, 134–50; process of, 7, 11–12, 14, 16–17, 28; prognosis for, 128–29, 140; risk factors for, 29–55, **30**; surgery for, 151–81; symptoms of, 56; terms for, 6–7; vascular inflammation and, 7, 11, 15–17, 22, 28, 38–41
Cough: ACE inhibitor-induced, 124–25; after surgery, 181
Coumadin, 95, 160
Cozaar (losartan), **123**
C-reactive protein, high-sensitivity (hs-CRP), 38–40, 92
Crestor (rosuvastatin), **35**
CT scanning, ultrafast, 61–64, **63**, 77
Cyclooxygenase (COX), 87
Cyclooxygenase 2 (COX2) inhibitors, 88–89
Cytochrome pathway, 94

Data and Safety Monitoring Board, 33, 111
Diabetes mellitus, 47–51, 182; adiponectin in, 48–49; angina in, 59;

High density lipoprotein (HDL), 11, 33, 35–36; altering relative amounts of LDL and, 36, 38; in diabetes, 48; function of, 36; raising level of, 36–38; smoking and, 53; transfer into LDL, 37
High-sensitivity C-reactive protein (hs-CRP), 38–40, 92
HIV from blood transfusion, 160
Hormone replacement therapy (HRT), 44–46
Hypertension, 51–52, 181–82; alpha-blocking drugs for, 112–13; kidney function and, 120–21; rebound, 113
Hytrin (terazosin), 113

Inderal (propranolol), 110–11, **110, 111**
Indigestion, 1, 18, 20, 56, 58, 74, 77, 84
Infarct expansion, 27
Infection: from blood transfusion, 160; postoperative, 161
Inflammation of arterial wall, 7, 11, 15–17, 22, 28, 38–41, 87
Informed consent for clinical trial participation, 33
Institutional Review Board, 33
Insulin, 47–49
Intensive care unit (ICU), 60, 155–56
Internal mammary artery grafts, **166,** 171–75, 178
Intracranial hemorrhage, 147
Ionic currents, 116
Irbesartan (Avapro), **123**
Isoptin (verapamil), **117**
Isosorbide dinitrate, 103
Isosorbide mononitrate, 103

Jump graft, 167

Kerlone (betaxolol), **110**
Kidney function: angiotensin II blockers and, 125; blood pressure and, 120–21

Labetalol (Normodyne), **110**
Laser-assisted angioplasty, 133
Left anterior descending coronary artery narrowing, 128–29, 140
Left circumflex artery narrowing, 128–29

Left internal mammary artery grafts, 171–75
Left main coronary artery disease, 128, 140
Lescol (fluvastatin), **35**
Levatol (penbutolol), **110**
Levine's sign, 58
Levitra (vardenafil), 102
Life expectancy, 3
Lifestyle changes, 51, 182–84
Lipid-laden macrophages, 16, 17, 22
Lipid Research Clinic Coronary Primary Prevention Trial (LRC-CPPT), 34, 97
Lipitor (atorvastatin), **35,** 92
Lipoprotein (a), 42
Lipoproteins, 10–11, 33, 41–43. *See also* High density lipoprotein; Low density lipoprotein
Lisinopril (Prinivil; Zestril), **123**
Liver injury, statin-induced, 94, **95**
Lopressor (metoprolol), **110**
Losartan (Cozaar), **123**
Lotensin (benazepril), **123**
Lovastatin (Mevacor), **35**
Low density lipoprotein (LDL), 11, 12; altering relative amounts of HDL and, 36, 38; CHD and, 16, 30; cholesterol transport via, 11, 14; in diabetes, 48; elevated hs-CRP and, 39; endothelial penetration by, 14–15; macrophages laden with, 16, 17, 22; medications for reduction of, 91–98; modified, 15; preventing absorption of, 33–34; protein composition of, 14–15; smoking and, 53; subintimal, 15

Macrophages, 15–16, 17, 22
Mavik (trandolapril), **123**
Mechanical ventilation, 153
Mediastinitis, postoperative, 161
Medications, 2, 12, 85–126; alpha-blocking drugs, 108–9, 112–13; beta-blocking drugs, 109–112, **110, 111;** for bypass graft disease, 169; calcium-channel-blocking drugs, 115–19, **117;** cholesterol-lowering, 91–98; combined alpha- and beta-blocking drugs, 114–15; epinephrine, 105, 106, 107; inhibitors of renin angiotensin

betic patients, 142–43, 144; for heart attack, 144–45, 147–49, **148**; *vs.* medications, 138–40; repetition of, 142–43; restenosis after, 135–36; subacute thrombosis and, 137–38

Percutaneous transluminal coronary angioplasty (PTCA), 130–33. *See also* Coronary angioplasty

Perindopril (Aceon), **123**

Persantine (dipyridamole), 75

Pharmacological stress test, 74–75

Phosphodiesterase inhibitors, 107

Physicians Health Study, 89

Pindolol (Visken), **110**

Placebo-controlled clinical trials, 32

Plaque. *See* Atherosclerotic plaque

Platelet inhibitors, 2, 86–91, 181; for angioplasty with stenting, 133, 137; for bypass graft disease, 169; for coronary bypass surgery, 167; preoperative, 160–61

Platelet plug, 87

Platelets, 23, 86–87, 91

Plavix (clopidogrel), 90–91, 178, 181; for angioplasty with stenting, 133, 137; preoperative, 160–61

Plendil (felodipine), **117**

Postmenopausal women, 43; HRT for, 44–46

PPAR modulators, 95–96

Pravastatin (Pravachol), **35**

Prazosin (Minipress), 112

Prinivil (lisinopril), **123**

Procardia (nifedipine), **117**

Progesterone, 43–45

Prognosis, 128–29, 140

Propranolol (Inderal), 110–11, **110, 111**

Prospective clinical trials, 32

Prostate enlargement, 113

Pseudoaneurysm, 83

Pulmonary embolus, 45

Pulse oximeter, 80

Questran (cholestyramine), 33–34, 97

Quinapril (Accupril), **123**

Radial artery grafts, 174–75

Radial Artery Patency Study (RAPS), 174–75

Radiation exposure, 62, 72

Ramipril (Altace), 122–24, **123**

Randomized clinical trials, 32

Ranolazine (Ranexa), 119–20

Remnant lipoproteins, 11

Renin angiotensin system, 121–25, **122**

Reperfusion therapy, 145–49; PCI, 147–49, **148**; thrombolytic agents, 145–47, **146**

Respirator, 153

Restenosis, 133; drug-eluting stents for prevention of, 135–36, 144; after stenting, 134–35

REVERSAL trial, 40, 92

Rhabdomyolysis, 93–94

Right coronary artery narrowing, 128–29

Right internal mammary artery grafts, 171–75

Risk factors, 29–55, **30**; aging, 29–30; cholesterol, 16, 30–38; diabetes mellitus, 47–51; elevated hs-CRP and vascular inflammation, 38–41; estrogen replacement, 43–46; genetic, 41–43; hypertension, 51–52; multiple, 53–55, **54**; smoking, 52–53

Risk reduction, 181–82

Robot-assisted coronary bypass surgery, 177–78

Rofecoxib (Vioxx), 88

Rosuvastatin (Crestor), **35**

Rotational atherectomy, 133

Saphenous vein graft, 164–71, 175; bypass graft disease in, 169–70; early thrombosis of, 167; jump, 167; loss of, 165–68; patency of, 165, **166**; repeat surgery after failure of, 170–71

Second messengers, 107

Sectral (acebutolol), **110**

Sequential bypass graft, 167

Shortness of breath, 20, 58, 66, 68

Sildenafil (Viagra), 102

Simvastatin (Zocor), **35**

Simvastatin/ezetimibe (Vytorin), 97

Sirolimus-eluting stents, 135–36

Smoking, 36, 52–53, 159, 169, 181, 182, 183–84

Smooth muscle cells, 16, 17, 22, 28

Society of Thoracic Surgeons, 157, 159

Statin agents, 2, 40–41, 48, 92–94, 181; for cholesterol reduction, 34–35, **35**, 92–95; after coronary bypass surgery, 169, 178; for hs-CRP reduction, 40; liver injury due to, 94, **95**; myopathy due to, 93–94

ST changes, exercise-induced, 66–67, **67**, 77

ST-elevation myocardial infarction, 23–24, 26, 124

Stent jail, 144

Stents, intracoronary, 133–40; in aging saphenous vein graft, 169; *vs.* coronary bypass surgery, 141–44; drug-eluting, 136–38, 143–44; *vs.* medications, 138–40; restenosis and, 134–35; risks of, 141; subacute thrombosis and, 137–38; success of, 134

Step-down unit, 156

Sternal incision, 154, 156; infection of, 161; postoperative care of, 179, 180; strength of, 179

Streptokinase, 145, 146, **146**

Stress-induced wall motion abnormality, 76–77

Stress test: abnormal, 77; exercise, 2, 63–69; with myocardial perfusion imaging, 70–75, **73**; pharmacological, 74–75; with wall motion analysis, 76–77

Stroke, 28, 30, 45, 124, 147, 175

Subacute thrombosis after stenting, 137–38

Sular (nisoldipine), **117**

Support hose, 181

Surgery. *See* Coronary bypass surgery

Sweating, 58

Sympathetic nervous system, 105, 179–80

Symptoms, 56–58

Synergy between PCI with Taxus and Cardiac Surgery (SYNTAX) trial, 144

Tadalafil (Cialis), 102

Tamsulosin (Flomax), 113

Tekturna (aliskiren), 125

Telmisartan (Micardis), **123**

Tenormin (atenolol), **110**

Terazosin (Hytrin), 113

Teveten (eprosartan), **123**

Thickening of arterial wall. *See* Arterial wall

Thrombolysis in Myocardial Infarction (TIMI) trials, 24

Thrombolytic therapy, 145–47, **146**; intracranial bleeding and, 147; *vs.* PCI, 147–49

Thrombophlebitis, 45

Thrombosis of venous bypass graft, 167

Thromboxane A2, 87

Thrombus formation, 23–24, 85, 132, 137. *See also* Blood clotting

Tiazac (diltiazem), **117**

Ticlopidine (Ticlid), 90

TIMI risk score, 24–26, **25**

Timolol (Blocadren), **110**

Tissue factor, 23

Tissue plasminogen activators, 145, 146

Toprol (metoprolol), **110**

Torcetrapib, 37

Tracheostomy, 153–54

Trandolapril (Mavik), **123**

Transesophageal echocardiogram, 163

Triglycerides, 48, 96

Trimetazidine, 119

Truncal obesity, 50

Turning Back the Clock Study, 183–84

Univasc (moexipril), **123**

Valdecoxib (Bextra), 88

Valsartan (Diovan), **123**

Vardenafil (Levitra), 102

Varicose veins, 164–65

Vascular inflammation, 7, 11, 15–17, 22, 28, 38–41, 87

Vasoconstriction, 99

Vasodilation, 19, 99–103

Vasotec (enalapril), **123**

Venous bypass grafts, 164–71; early thrombosis of, 167; jump, 167; loss of, 165–68, 165–69; patency of, 165, **166**; quality of veins for, 164–65; repeat surgery after failure of, 170–71; treating bypass graft disease in, 169–70

Ventilator, 153

Verapamil (Calan; Isoptin), **117**
Very light density lipoprotein (VLDL), 11
Viagra (sildenafil), 102
Vioxx (rofecoxib), 88
Visken (pindolol), **110**
Vitamin B6, 36, 96
Vytorin (simvastatin/ezetimibe), 97

Walking after surgery, 180
Weight loss: to reduce diabetes risk, 51; after surgery, 157, 180

Women's Health Initiative (WHI), 45–46

X-rays, 61, 78

Zebeta (bisoprolol), **110**
Zestril (lisinopril), **123**
Zetia (ezetimibe), 97
Zocor (simvastatin), **35**

Disclosure

Within the past five years, the author has received financial support in the form of speaker's honoraria or consulting fees from the following companies:

Datascope Inc., Cardiac Assist Division
Edwards Life Sciences LLC
Johnson & Johnson Inc., Cordis Division
Merck Inc.
Millennium Pharmaceuticals Inc.
Novartis Inc.